The Holistic House

A sanctuary for health and wellbeing

Jean-Marie Gobet

How should a house be built so that it acts as an agent of transformation and inspiration for the human soul? Can such a house be built?

The architect-priests of ancient Egypt not only believed buildings should embody our social values and individual tastes but strived for them to have their own soul. They used this knowledge and wisdom to erect temples and public buildings, a knowledge that architect Jean-Marie Gobet spreads and shares through his latest book (The Holistic House - A sanctuary for health and wellbeing).

We have the knowledge and ability to not simply build houses that will benefit our health but to promote our spiritual, emotional and physical evolution.

CONTENTS

01 /
Introduction

Have you ever found your child curled up in a corner of the bed? Have you ever noticed that your cat chooses particular spots to sleep? Does your dog seem to deliberately avoid certain areas? Do you feel more comfortable in certain parts of your home than others? Are you affected by recurrent migraines, allergies or insomnia you cannot explain?

DEFINITION OF GEOBIOLOGY

Have you ever found your child curled up in a corner of the bed? Have you ever noticed that your cat chooses specific spots to sleep? Does your dog seem to deliberately avoid certain areas? Do you feel more comfortable in certain parts of your home than others? Are you affected by recurrent migraines, allergies or insomnia you cannot explain?

As I progressed through my studies in architecture, I became frustrated at my inability to express my feelings and my insights about such questions because they were not understood by mainstream architecture.

Most people can express their opinion about a site, a house or a specific living space. Comments such as "This place gives me the creeps" or "I feel so good in this room" are obvious realities to the people who express them. They are based on our innate ability to appreciate what is beneficial or detrimental to our well-being. Strangely these realities are usually not included in the design process as valid decision criteria. Since they cannot be rationally explained, they are quickly dismissed.

Geobiology suggests answers to questions like these. It strives to analyse age old building traditions and to support them with recent discoveries of science. The term geobiology originates from the Greek words Geos (earth), Bios (life) and Logos (discourse). It includes the study of the radiations that traverse the Earth, radiations that ultimately constitute the energy that animates our Mother Earth, which can be considered a living being with a skeleton of rocks, a nourishing liquid in the form of water, and a nervous system whose paths, like Chinese meridians, convey telluric energy from the cosmos. These radiations influence the life and health of living beings.

This knowledge of telluric energies by humans is not a recent discovery; it was known as Geomancy in ancient times. The study of the placement of megaliths and numerous temples proves that for millennia, humans have been able to construct certain monuments considering the forces of the earth. While the knowledge of telluric radiations seems to date to ancient times, its designation under the term Geobiology is relatively recent.

With the growth of industrialisation and the rapid changes in construction methods, problems associated with geopathic stress and sick building syndrome started to be more frequents. This gave rise to greater awareness about the quality living space. Baubiologie emerged in the 1960s in Germany as a response to growing concerns about the impact of buildings on human health and the environment, emphasizing a holistic approach to building design and construction. While in France and Switzerland the same problems brought to the fore Geobiology which examines the relationship between the local environment and the health of living organisms by integrating the studies and the discoveries of many specialised fields such as physics, geophysics, geology, hydrology, biology, electronics, architecture and tradition both local and collective.

8

THE NEED FOR A NEW WAY OF BUILDING

1 James Lovelock - Gaia,
The Practical Science of Planetary Medicine
1991

When society moved into the industrial age, an entire body of knowledge, accumulated through centuries of studies and observation was suddenly disregarded. The art of building was deprived of its sacred aspects and its rituals. It had become a purely materialistic endeavour in a materialistic world.

Every civilisation, every tradition that preceded us took for granted the fact that man was part of a greater whole and that his was a key role in the interplay of natural forces. Humanity saw itself as the vessel in which the cosmic energies and the earthly energies where transmuted for the purpose of its evolution. The buildings erected by pre-industrial societies supported man in his great task, to spiritualize matter and to materialise spirit.

What are the temples and cathedrals of today? They are the banks, insurance company headquarters, shopping centres, structures which, more often than not, adversely affect the health of their occupants.

Cities and suburbs are planned by technicians mostly concerned with traffic flow, the power distribution grid and commercial land values. The fact a residential development could be built in an unsuitable geological area or even on land that has been used for chemical waste dumping is often consciously disregarded.

Traditionally the act of choosing a town site was surrounded by a set of rituals through which the site would reveal its ability to hold human activities.

In his -Ten Books on Architecture- the Roman architect Vitruvius Pollio explained how the site for a new city was chosen, cattle were to be left grazing on the land for a year and then slaughtered. Their entrails were then examined and only after their state of good health was confirmed would the site be declared sound and healthy.

Our houses are the crystallisation of society's ideas, the materialisation of our values, and the embodiment of our knowledge of the world. As we pour concrete into the formwork, we pour our view of the world.

As our ideas, values and knowledge change so must our constructions, and, as we become wiser and more enlightened so must our work.

During the last 200 years, our species has systematically destroyed, poisoned and polluted our environment, first the urban centres and more recently the whole planet. This process is felt by most of us. Some new solutions such as Geobiology (from the Greek Ge, the earth; Bios, life; Logos, study) were studied and proposed to relieve some of the problems inherent to industrial development.

What Geobiology proposes is a new and unique way to interact with our environment, mainly in the field of town planning and construction. This original approach is characterised by a new awareness, a new awakening and a new way of looking at the land born of a vision of the Earth as being a living self-sustaining organism as described by James Lovelock in his book, Gaia, The Practical Science of Planetary Medicine, where he sees the earth as:

"A single physiological system, an entity that is alive at least to the extent that, like other living organisms, its chemistry and temperature are self-regulating at a state favourable for life."[1]

Apart from avoiding the obvious senseless and thoughtless rape of the site prior to building haphazardly on its scarred surface geobiology will promote a gentle awakening or crystallisation of the inherent potential of the site. It will bring out the pre-existing blueprint of its purpose. Man will then be the instrument of materialisation in tune with nature.

The land will lovingly nestle a habitat which will, at first glance, show humanity' respect for beauty and nature, and exude a sense of peaceful contentment. The home will regenerate its

9

inhabitants. It will be a place where people will love to come and stay, a place where they will feel deep within themselves the love of the universe for mankind. The vibrations will be uplifting.

Within the field of geobiological studies the age old native and local traditions of respect for the land and modern technologies are married for the specific purpose of offering a habitat that is more than just a shelter but will give people a sweeping view of who they are through the symbolic level down to the physical level. It will seem like the community was always there, belonging there from eternity, born of this very site after a long gestation.

The purpose is not to merely design and build a habitat that is located on a healthy site, without geopathic stress and free of toxic material, but to use our knowledge to make our dwelling the instrument to raise our energy and consciousness.

Cities and suburbs are planned by technicians mostly concerned by traffic flow, the power distribution grid and commercial land values.

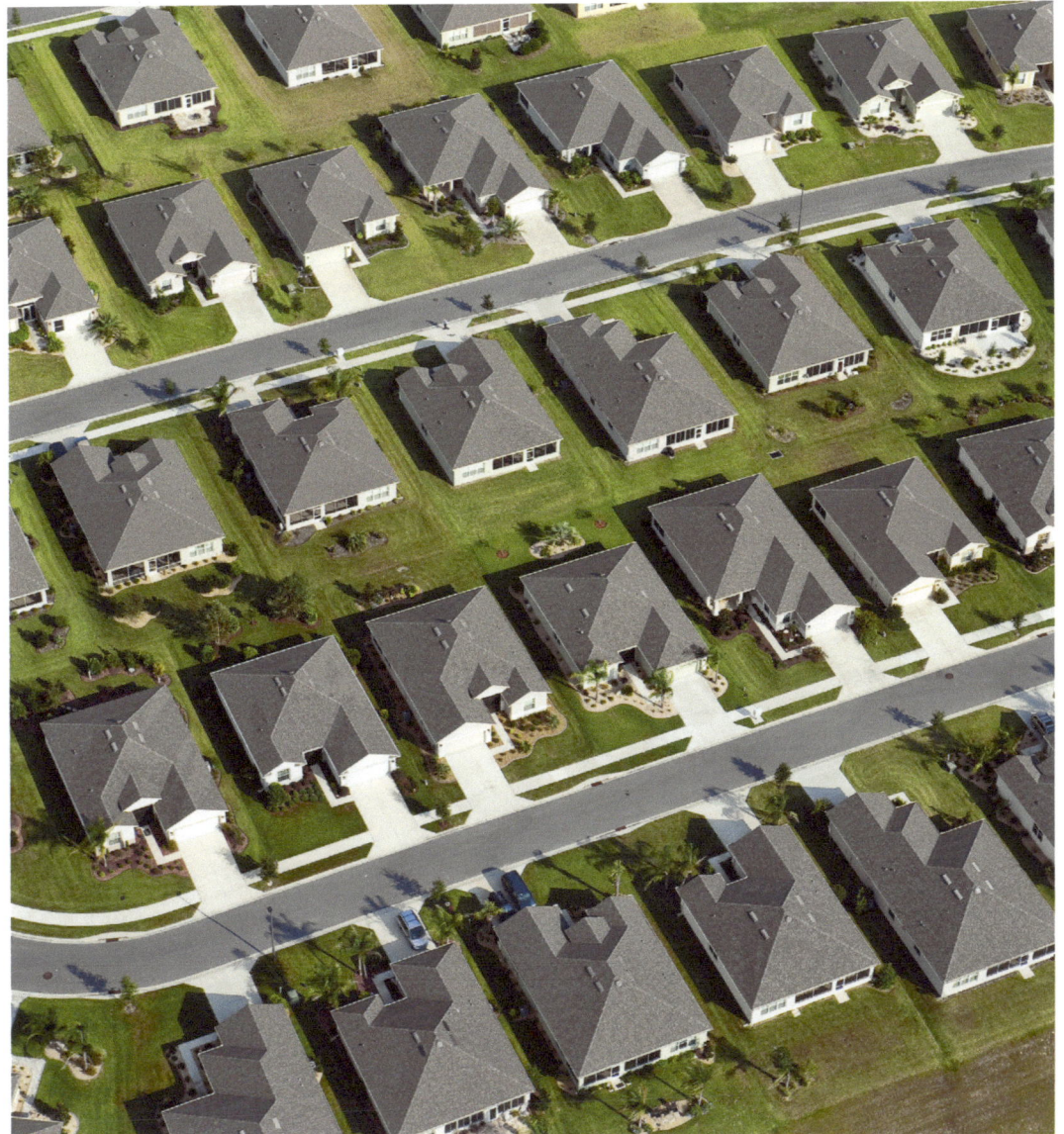

10

THE STRUCTURE OF GEOBIOLOGY

Geobiology aims to provide the information for us to reproduce a habitat as near to natural living conditions as possible, giving consideration to the need for comfort provided by ancient and new technologies favourable to the environment. It strives to define and examine the numerous elements influencing the quality of our home. To diminish or enhance the health of the house many elements need to come together which we can order into three interdependent categories, or levels.

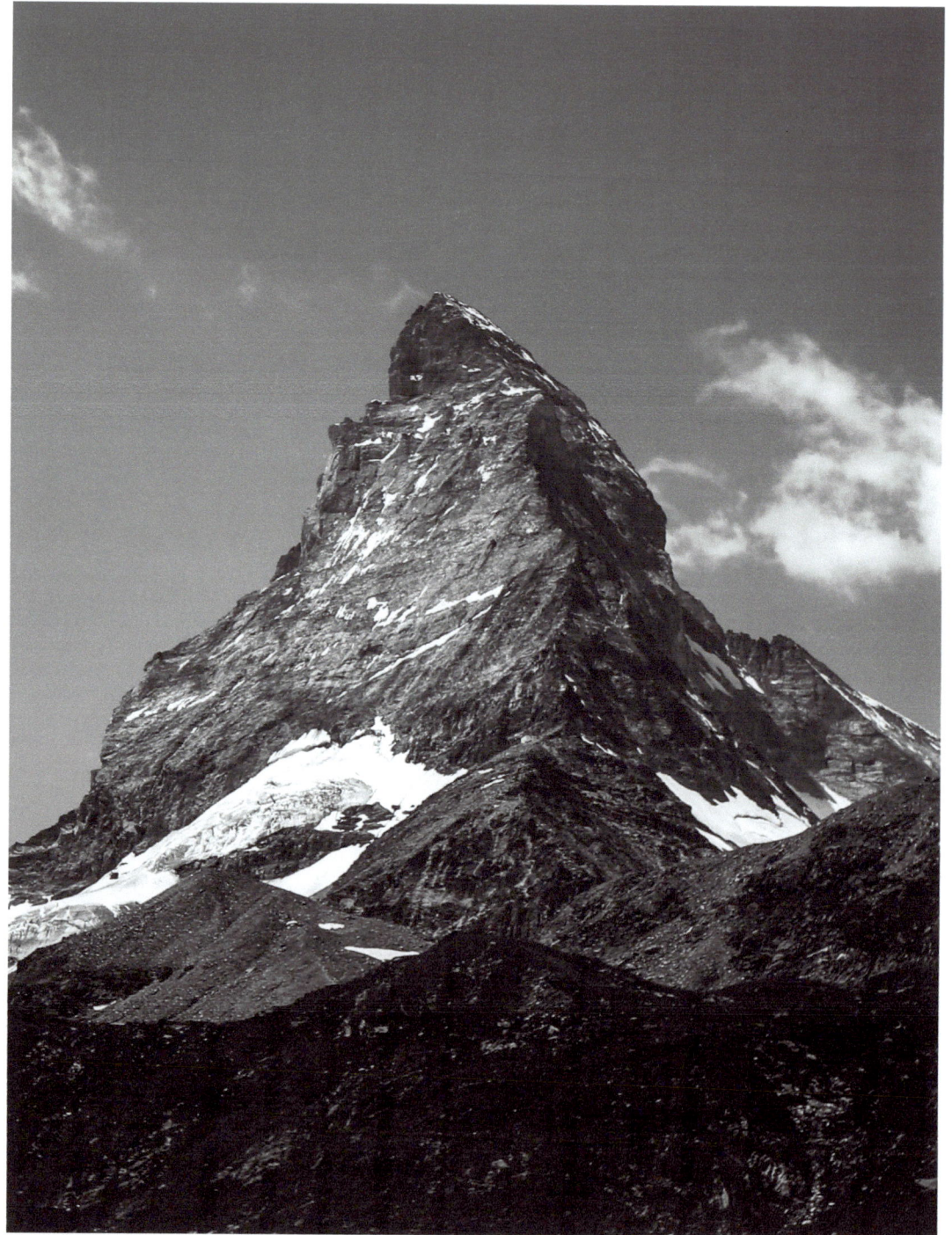

Matterhorn

PHYSICAL LEVEL

The physical level deals with all the known effects related to the quality of the ground -such as geological faults, underground water streams, radon gas emanations- to the quality of the location. This includes -ground, water and air pollution, and the quality of construction (nontoxic building materials and nontoxic paints).

We have slowly come to realise the profound influence building materials have on our health, both physical and psychological. You can easily imagine yourself holding a piece of wood, feeling its softness and warmth. The tree has grown drawing its energy from each element, earth, water, air and the sun. The wood radiates a message of life, very different to the feeling of touching a piece of polystyrene or a piece of plastic. But even the best materials can be killed by toxic chemical treatments which are slowly releasing poisonous emanations such as lead, cadmium, formaldehyde, phenol and organochlorins. They are known to cause nausea, headaches, insomnia, asthma, brain damage and even cancer.

ENERGY LEVEL

The energy level includes the positioning of the house on the Hartmann grid and other tellurian currents, electromagnetic pollution and the Faraday cage effect due to bad earthing of electric installations, reinforcement of concrete slabs and steel frames.

In recent years, the rapid proliferation of artificial sources of radio-electrical frequencies has become a cause for concern. It has surpassed many times the production of natural sources. According to a German specialist, Dr. Wolfgang Volkrodt, electromagnetic pollution has increased a hundredfold during the past 50 years.

Ten to fifteen per cent of cancers affecting American children could be caused by low frequency electromagnetic fields around high voltage power lines. This is the astonishing affirmation of the "New York Power Lines Project".

This study group was formed by the commission responsible for the power grid of the State of New York.

SYMBOLIC LEVEL

The symbolic or spiritual level, which is the least recognised, is also the most important because it defines the quality of the whole. Most of us can clearly feel the difference of ambience in extremes -for example between abattoirs and churches- and be strongly affected by them. Persons endowed with a greater sensitivity will perceive subtle differences that would nevertheless influence us unconsciously. According to Blanche Merz (Institute of Geobiology of Chardonne, Switzerland) just as a place can make us prone to disease or depression, another can lift us to more subtle levels of vibration, strengthening our body and spirit. Such places were sought throughout history and held as sacred.

Some are natural wonders like Uluru, the Grand Canyon, the Matterhorn and countless other places on this planet which inspire the millions of modern pilgrims we call tourists.

Others are manmade poles of attraction built on powerful sites by architect-priests obeying a sacred tradition, like the pyramids of Egypt, the statues of Easter Island or many Gothic cathedrals. The site of the Chartres cathedral in France was already considered sacred by the Celts.

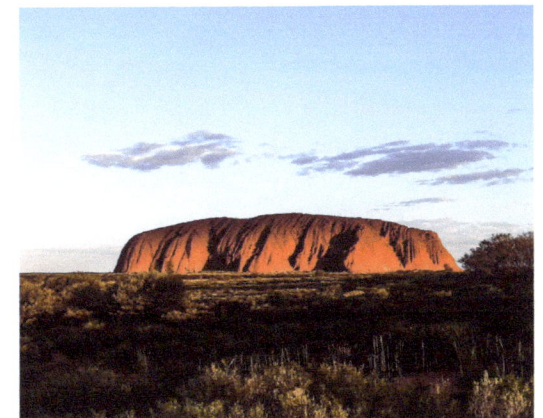

Uluru

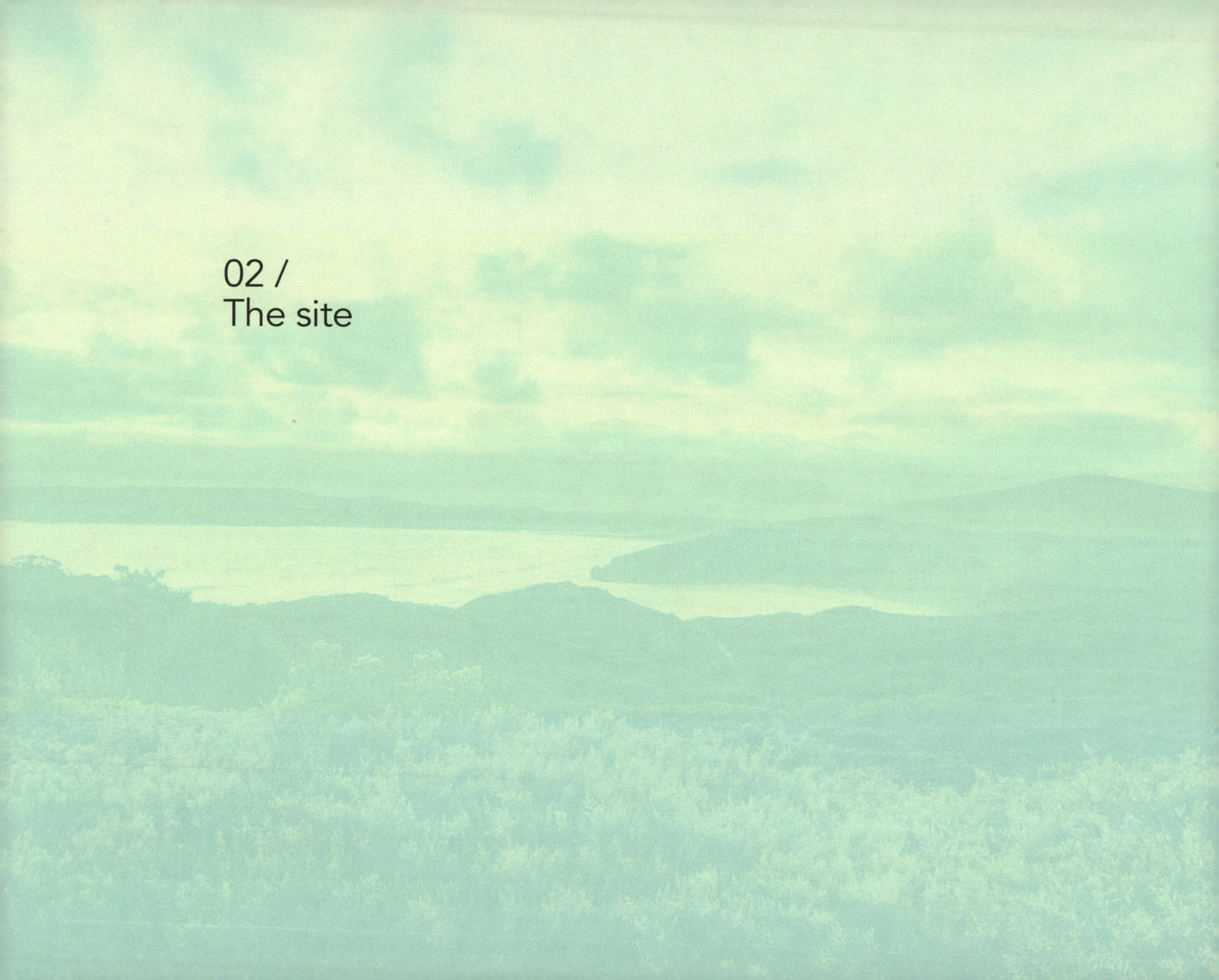

02 /
The site

13

SITE READING

One can get lost in the techniques, forgetting the feelings generated by finer perceptions of the environment. We do not trust ourselves.
When approaching a site, all our senses should be open and receptive to what is around. But the main focus of our awareness should be placed on ourselves, on our reactions to this sensory input. These reactions are the standard by which we determine the quality of our connection to a particular site.

BETWEEN EARTH AND HEAVENS

A healthy house should not cut its inhabitant from the natural influences of heaven and earth. It should be the haven where one can regenerate. To achieve this construction must keep as much of the original natural radiation of the environment as possible.

Humanity has evolved within this field of radiation for over 40000 generations and has developed a highly sensitive nervous system. Modern technology and new housing techniques have deprived us of contact with nature after only three or four generations. There has been little time for biological adaptation. This field of energies is often called "Cosmo-tellurian forces". It implies the combination of both the energies of heaven (cosmos) and of the Earth (tellus in Latin).

INFLUENCES OF THE EARTH

The geomagnetic field

The influences generated by the Earth are generally from the Earth's magnetic field and local geological characteristics. Our planet behaves as an enormous magnet with its positive (North) and negative (South) poles surrounded by its own magnetic field (the geomagnetic field) pulsating at the rate of 7.8 beats per second, it is the strongest of all the planets. This field is so important as to have been artificially induced

in space stations for the wellbeing of the occupants.

Geological studies show that through time the magnetic field has shifted This can be seen in ancient volcanic rocks, as they "crystallised" in alignment with the existing magnetic field.

The study of residual magnetism in rock formations shows that the magnetic field of the Earth has reversed its polarity as many as 170 times in the last 100 million years.

The spiral shaped snail shells are known to have changed their sense of rotation after a reversal of polarity of the geomagnetic field.

The position of the magnetic poles changes noticeably from year to year, measurements of this change shows that the whole magnetic field is drifting westwards up to 24 km per annum.

When a piece of rock is placed on a slab of cork and floated on still water it will align itself with the magnetic field of the Earth, according to its own polarity.

The intensity of the geomagnetic field is not constant; its intensity is affected by numerous factors such as the latitude of the site, its altitude, solar activity, the Earth's rotation speed and the magnetic pole's continual shift. The daily variations of the magnetic field present

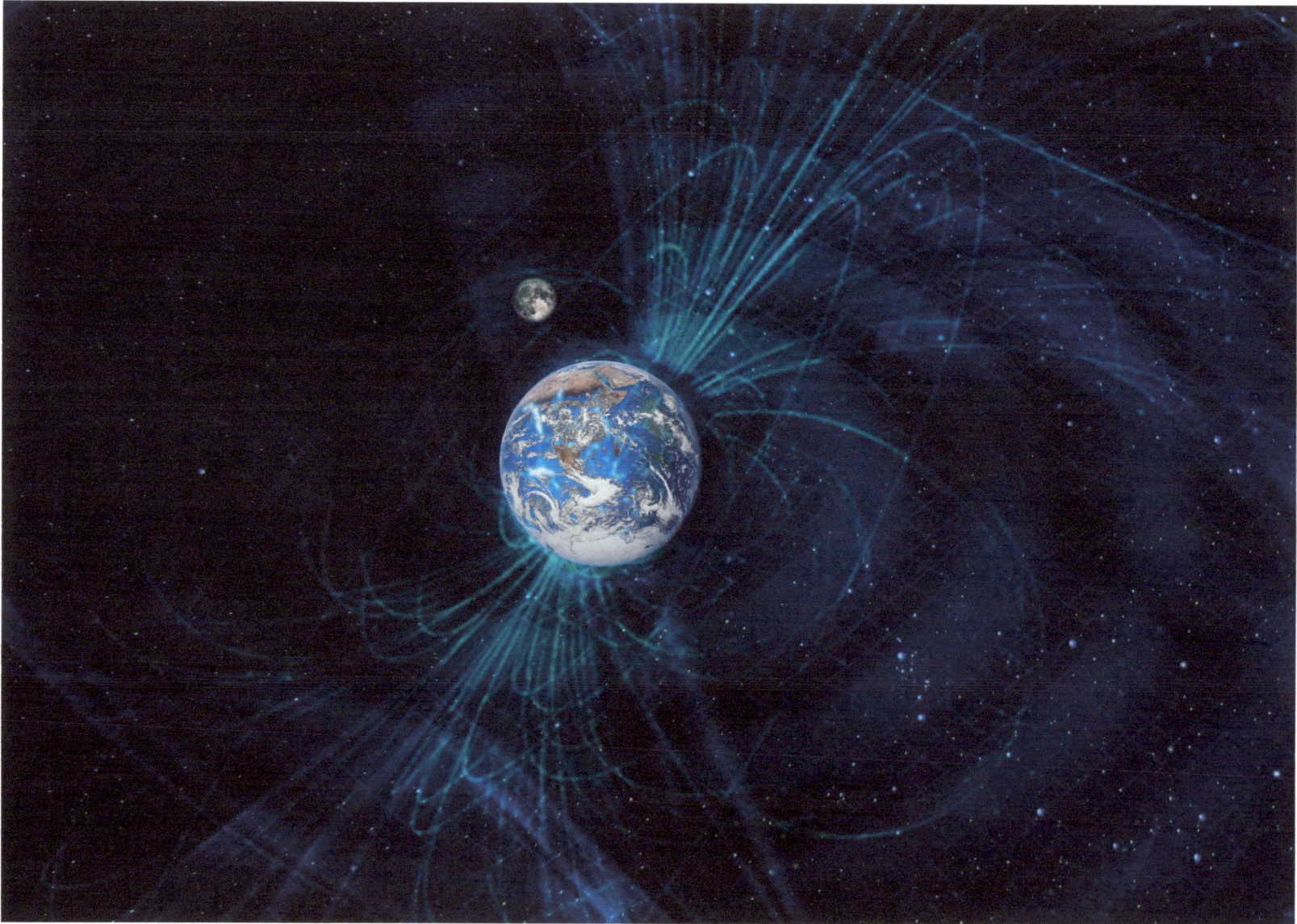

15

2 Georges Lakhovsky
(The Secret of Life)
Tri State Press

3 Georges Lakhovsky
(The Secret of Life)
Tri State Press

two lows and two highs, one of the low points is around 4 o'clock in the morning, the hour when most insomniacs finally fall asleep.

The magnetic field is also affected by the ground's geological structure such as geological faults and water-veins above which one can observe pulsating fields.

Geometrical shapes, -linear, two or three dimensional-, receive this magnetic radiation, transform it and transmit it with more or less intensity.

Geological aspects

The father of western medicine, the Greek physician Hippocrates (460-375 BC) was one of the first to study the connection between health and habitat. Sedentary man lives under the direct influence of the local climate and the physical, chemical, geological and magnetic nature of the ground. The local soil conditions will also affect him indirectly through the water he drinks, and the quality of the food grown locally. Some are conducive to a harmonious life and others to diseases.

People living in areas where the water or the soil is poor in calcium will suffer from brittle bones (rickets). If on the other hand there is a surplus of calcium they will be prone to bladder problem due to calculus (kidney stones).

The lack of iodine in certain areas such as the Alps in Europe or the Great Lakes region and inland mountains in the U.S, will cause the development of goitre, an enlargement of the thyroid gland. Children born with thyroxin deficiency (secreted by the thyroid) will be characterised by a defective mental and physical development called cretinism.

Recurring fevers often affect populations living where clay is found over volcanic rock formations.

A thorough geobiological survey requires a good knowledge of the geological nature of the surroundings as well as an understanding of the site itself. It will thus be easier to explain the diverse phenomena that have been observed.

According to the studies of Georges Lakhovsy[2] *"Analysis shows that low cancer densities (0.5 - 0.8 per 1000 inhabitants) coincide with a vast area of sand and sandstone in Beauchamp in the Paris Basin.*

On the other hand, we see the district where cancer density is high, such as Auteuil (1.76), Javel (1.61), Grenelle (2.08) and Saint Lambert (1.57) rest on plastic clay. Other district such as Saint-Vincent -de-Paul (1.97), L'Hopital Saint Louis (1.44), Pere Lachaise (1.58) and Charonne (1.41) are situated on marly soils."

In a comparable study published in 1875 English Doctor Alfred Haviland brought to the notice of the medical profession the following results:[3]

- The districts which had the lowest mortality from cancer were characterised geologically by the older (Palaeozoic) and most elevated rocks, such as the Lower and Carboniferous Limestone series: and by the secondary (Mesozoic) Limestone of the Oolites as well as chalk formations.

- The districts which had the highest mortality were characterised geologically by clays, such as the London clay of the Eocene, the Boulder clay of the Pleistocene or Glacial period, and the brick earths and alluvial deposits of recent origin.

COSMIC INFLUENCES

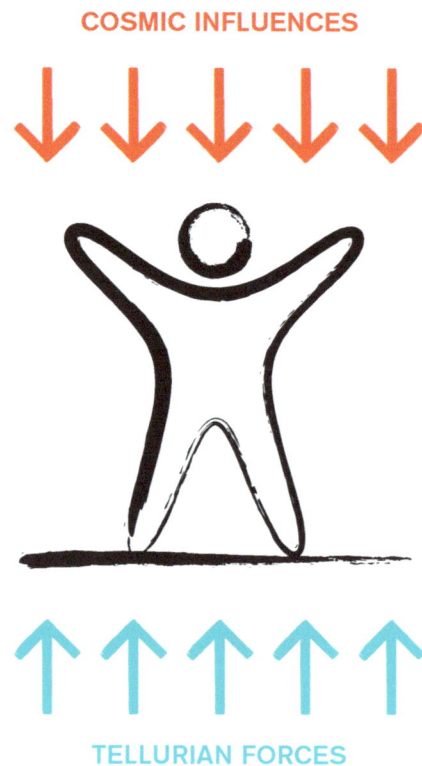

TELLURIAN FORCES

COSMIC INFLUENCES

The Sun

The Sun is undoubtedly the greatest cosmic influence on the surface of our planet. It is the giver if life and many civilisations have made it the symbol of God's presence in our universe. Apart from light, heat, and electromagnetic radiation covering nearly six octaves, it also generates rays similar to X-rays and waves comparable to radio waves. The solar radiation reaches the earth in eight minutes and most of it is stopped in the upper layers of the atmosphere.

Medical science tells us that the effect of solar radiation on our organism is as follow:

- Certain skin bacteria are destroyed

- The skin secretes immunising substances protecting against infectious diseases

- The number of white cells is increased

- The blood produces substances having a toning effect on our muscles

- Our body produces vitamin D

- The development of hormones is stimulated

- With the penetration of U.V. rays (0,25 wave length) veins will dilate and blood circulation is stimulated

In the 17th century the first observation of solar activity was made with the discovery of sunspots. It became understood that our star is an evolving living body.

Solar activity includes also flare jets of gas and matter shooting as high as 4000 km from the surface of the sun.

These eruptions are accompanied by great disruption of the magnetic field, radio waves, X-radiation and particles which sometimes disrupt radio communication on Earth and generate northern lights, "aurora borealis".

The increase and decrease of sunspots activity follow an 11-year cycle. Many observations have been made about the probable influence of these 11-year cycles they have been connected to the seismic and volcanic activity of our planet, the production of wheat, the quality of certain vintages for wine, historical and sociological events.

In the highest level of our atmosphere gas molecules are maintained by solar radiation forming a zone called ionosphere. The properties of the ionosphere are subjected to daily and seasonal variations, as well as variations induced by the sunspots activity. Certain radio waves travel better at night than during the day and better in December than in June. The movement of particles travelling along the Sun's magnetic field generates solar wind and can

17

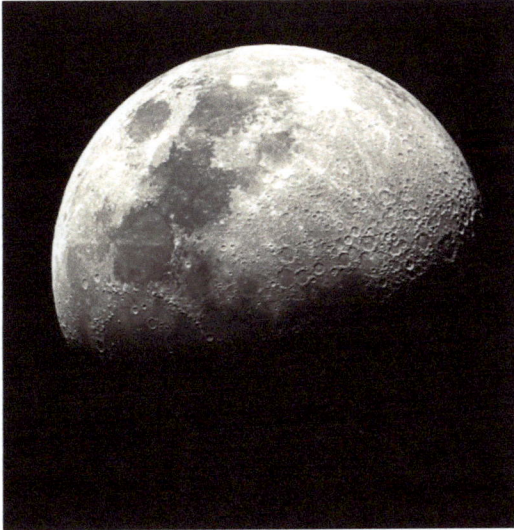

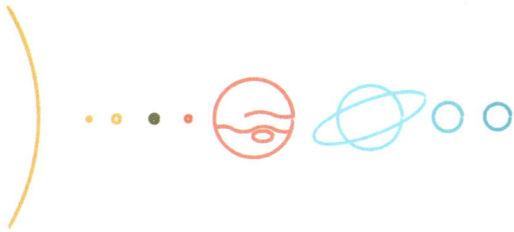

cause disturbances detectable in the Earth's magnetic field.

The Moon

The Earth satellite is the celestial body nearest to us. From the beginning of time its regular 29,5 days cycle has determined the movement of tides, both oceanic and terrestrial. It is less known that the lithosphere, the rocky crust of the earth, can move up to 50cm at high tide. The geomagnetic field can vary according to the day and the lunar month. The relation between certain phases of the Moon and periods of intense rain has been scientifically observed.

The lunar cycles affect everything from the surface of our planet to the most inner core of our psyche. Many gardeners and farmers still follow the Moon for planting and harvesting. The lunar cycle is also said to affect women's menstrual cycle. Full Moon nights are also known to affect the number of road accidents. Rodents that have been completely isolated are still affected by the lunar cycles.

In the Swiss Alps, it is the custom to light the first fire in a new or newly renovated chimney only when the Moon is full or waxing. If the fire was to be lit at the waning Moon, it is thought the chimney would never draw properly. On the other hand, construction wood was traditionally only felled when the Moon is waning between the months of December and February. When the sap would be at its lowest.

The Planets and the Stars

Jupiter, Venus and Saturn send us their radiation as well. Jupiter radiates almost twice as much energy as it receives from the Sun, its radio electrical waves output is the most important in the solar system after the Sun.

Radio astronomy has enabled us to discover other sources of radiation in the cosmos such as stars (novae and supernovas), quasars and pulsars, even from distant galaxies. In March 1951 radiation from a hydrogen cloud. The most common element in the Universe was detected, this discovery enabled us to calculate the hydrogen atom emission wavelength (21cm).

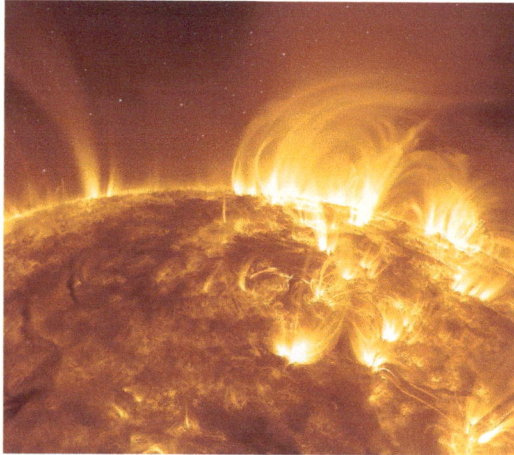

Disturbances in the magnetosphere caused by solar winds.

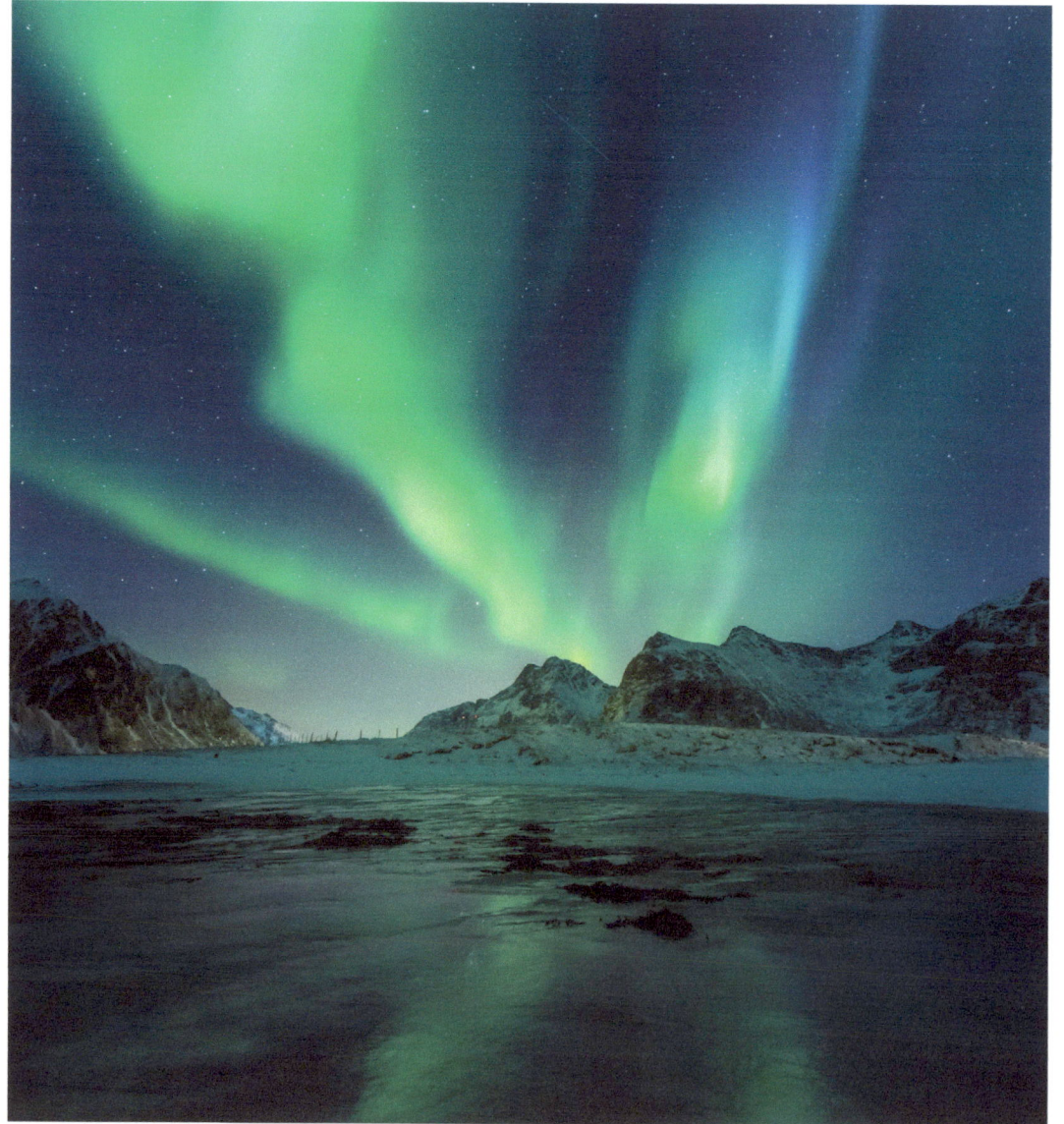

19

INTERRACTION OF COSMO-TELLURIAN FORCES

4 Rudolf Steiner (Anthroposophy and Science)

As we have seen above, we are subjected to the influence of two main categories of forces - cosmic forces and tellurian forces. When these energies are in harmony man becomes the vessel in which these forces are transmuted for his physical, psychological and spiritual wellbeing. Since there is no perfect site on this planet, man has evolved designs, building techniques and ways of defining the quality of the site to harmonise these energies.

One way to look at it is that the cosmic forces which are continuously showering us have the purpose of neutralising the tellurian forces. The interaction between these forces is known as the Cosmo-tellurian field. The subtle harmony of this field can be disturbed by several factors.

According to Rudolf Steiner[4], *tellurian forces express their essence in an ascending movement and could be represented by two hands joined in prayer and architecturally by the Gothic arch. As for cosmic forces, their downwards movement is symbolised by both hands open, palms towards the sky in a receptive gesture which is translated architecturally by a column's capital.*

Atmosphere and electricity

As the Sun radiates ultraviolet rays and showers electrons, it ionises certain layers of the atmosphere causing them to conduct electricity. Atmospheric electricity is also generated by movements of clouds of ions carried by atmospheric tides. These tides are the result of solar and lunar interaction on the Earth atmosphere.

The difference of potential between the cosmos and the surface of the Earth is about 0.0078 volt. The Earth is acting as the negative element of a gigantic condenser of which the cosmos is the positive element. From the surface of the Earth to the ionosphere the tension rises to 400,000 volts, an average of 100 volts per metre of height difference. For a human being of average height, it represents a difference of 170 volts while standing, this is reduced to almost nothing while lying down, to rest or sleep for example.

Our body is like an antenna capturing the electrical signals of the environment and our metabolism follows these daily cycles. Maximum electricity occurs around 8 p.m. (high blood pressure) and the minimum around 4 a.m. (low blood pressure). The intensity of this cycle is modified by seasonal changes with the level of electricity higher in summer than in winter.

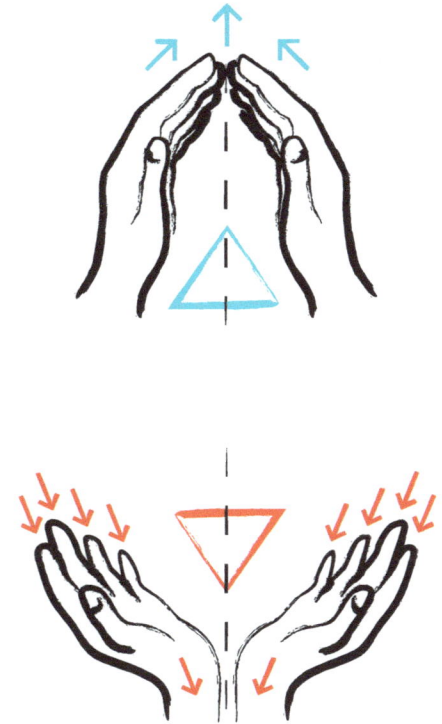

20

Ionisation of the air

The regenerating property of the air is directly proportional to its content in negative ions. It has been found that negative ions have a strong influence on the vitality and the health of living organisms.

Positive and negative ions are present in the atmosphere in roughly equal numbers. They are produced by shortwave radiation hitting gas molecules, generating positive ions lacking an electron and negative ions holding one electron too many. An atom is naturally stable when its positive and negative charges are balanced; this is why negative and positive ions are short lived.

The positive ions quickly regain stability by -stealing- electrons from the environment, especially living organisms, slowly depleting them of their energy.

On the other hand, the negative ions give energy by shedding their superfluous electron.

Negatively charged ions are depleted by polluted, smoky, dry air, by electrical fields and by static from synthetic carpets and fabrics. The weather also plays a role in altering the quantity of negative ions when hot dry winds blow, or before a storm. Negative ions can be produced by plants and trees and moving water, such as creeks, waterfalls and rainstorms.

Geological nature of the ground

The reaction of the ground to cosmic radiation depends on the geological nature of the site, if it is a bad conductor of electricity such as sand or gravel, the radiation propagates without being absorbed, or if there is absorption it is weak and in such a wide volume that the reaction on the surface is hardly perceptible. On the other hand, when the ground is a good conductor of electricity -clay, iron ore- the radiation is rapidly absorbed on the surface and creates a disturbance as it is reflected, deflected and diffracted.

The ground can be thus classified in two main categories defined by good conductivity and bad conductivity; the former can modify the harmony and the vibration rate of the cells and facilitate the development of cancer.

These electrical fields are not stable and homogenous, they can be influenced by the conductivity of the ground, animals and plants can inform us about the nature of the electrical charge, whether positive, neutral or negative.

Radon gas

The ground can be the cause of radioactive pollution when it is the source of radon gas emanation. This odourless and colourless gas is the result of the disintegration of uranium or granitic based rock formations. It seeps through dry geological faults and finds its way

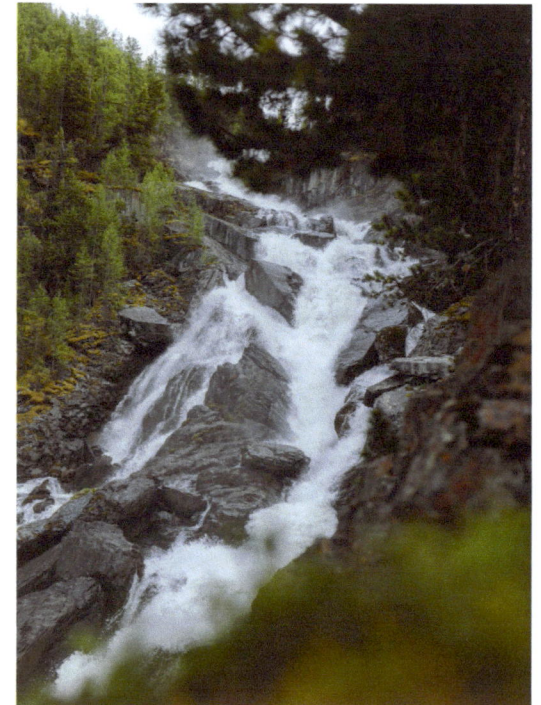

21

Often, trees growing above water-veins or geological faults will present defects and growths.

5 Robert Endros (Le rayonnement de la terre et son influence sur la vie) Signal

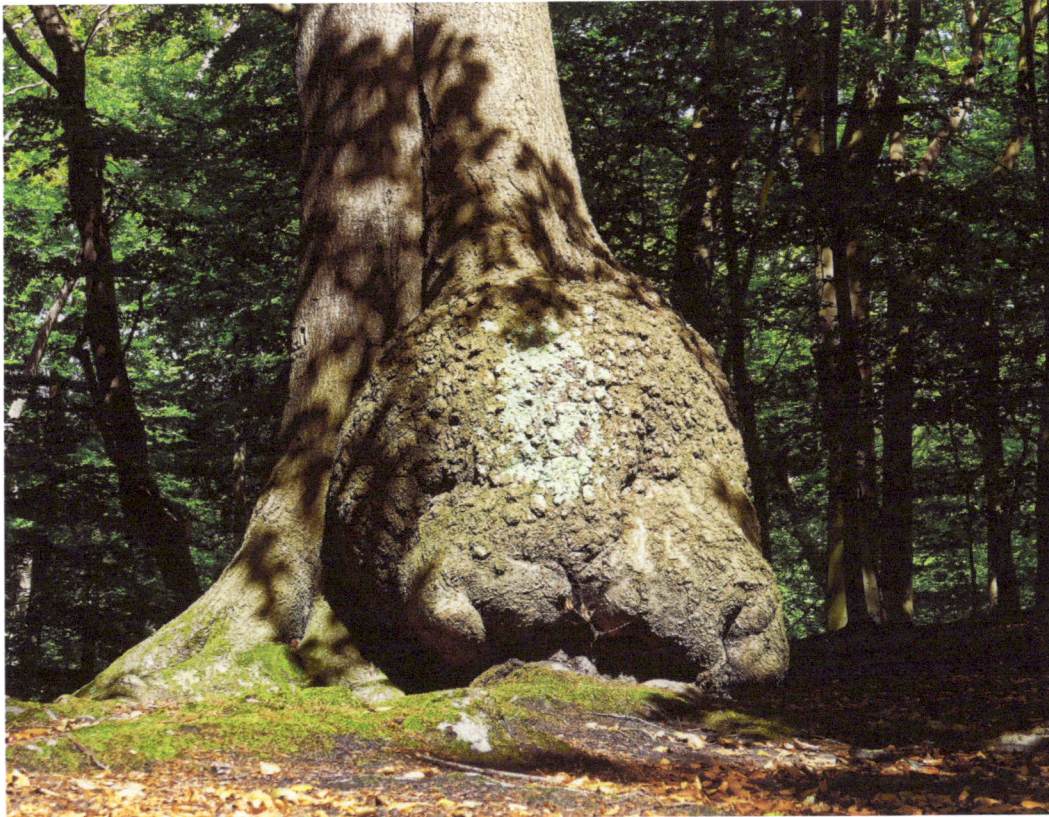
Deformed tree trunk growing on a water vein.

through canalisation pipes, concrete slabs, stones and brick walls. It accumulates in cellars and other areas that are poorly ventilated; it can then accumulate to dangerous levels, up to many hundred times higher than outside.

It is wise to study the nature of the ground before building and to consult the local health department to know the radon level in a given area.

Houses built on sensitive areas, that are used only over week ends or holidays can accumulate a high concentration of radon gas.

Some simple construction technique can be used to keep the level of radon below dangerous levels. It can be a sealed waterproof membrane under the concrete slab. But the best solution is a ventilated space between the ground and the living space.

Animals and plants

Throughout history animals have constituted the economic base of rural properties and the greatest care has been taken to build healthy shelters for them. We rarely see old farm buildings situated on a disturbed area. Most of the cases of diseased animals observed by Professor Endros[5] living over geopathic zones have been observed in installations built in recent decades.

Horse breeders who have worked for many generations on the same property have noticed through experience that every horse that has been put in a particular box becomes nervous and loses weight. Sometimes they are even affected by dermatitis and when racing the results are badly affected. Calves, chickens and pigs are also very sensitive.

22

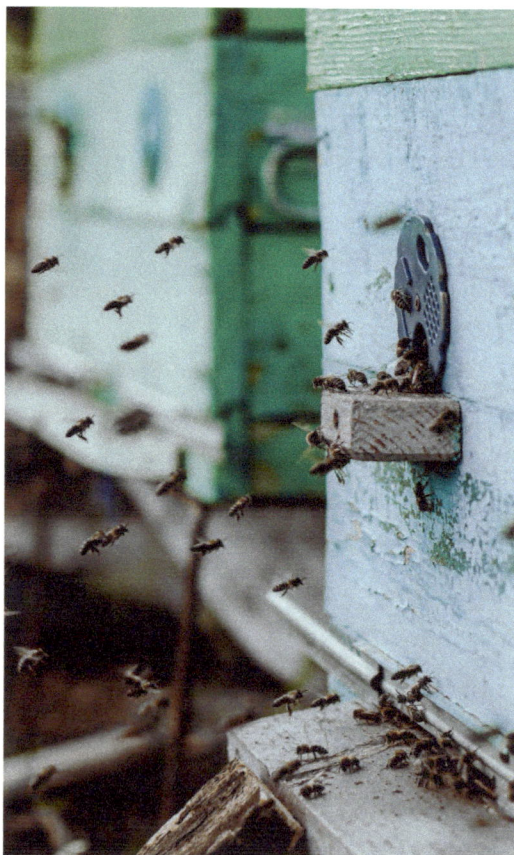

6 Dr. Quinquandon
(12 Balles pour un
Veto) Agriculture
et vie

It is interesting to note that cats, snails, slugs and salamanders will thrive over negative zones but dogs, chickens, ducks and quails like positive zones. As for asparagus, ants, flies, rabbits and mice neutral zones are preferred.

In the 1930s, Dr S. Jenny of Aarau in (Switzerland) experimented with the effect of radiation generated by geological faults and underground streams on 25,000 mice over a period of 12 years. Mice in cages placed over an irregularity of the geomagnetic field became agitated, gnawed their tails and even ate their offspring. Sometimes they developed cancerous tumours. When placed over a neutral zone they became more settled. If a cage was placed partly over such a disturbance and partly on a healthy zone the mice preferred to stay on the latter, where they would also always choose to give birth.

Often, trees growing above water-veins or geological faults will present defects and growths.

In France, some beekeepers place hives over underground water veins. Such hives can produce up to three times more honey than hives positioned a few feet away. According to these beekeepers, the life span of these bees is considerably shortened and they are more aggressive. The hives are placed over a neutral area to rest during winter.

According to Dr Henry Quinquandon[6], a French veterinarian, who has observed many animals on geopathic zones, the symptoms are usually typical to each species.

- Rabbits lose their hair. Dogs suffer from arthritis.

- Chickens lose weight and can die of leukaemia.

- Pigs are affected by liver and blood diseases Horses might be affected by heart diseases, arthritis, eczema, loss of hair and blindness.

- Cattle will show a considerable decrease of milk production and even sterility. Sheep are affected by liver diseases.

Human beings:

With human beings, certain recurrent health problems can be attributed to geopathic stress, especially when a tried and trusted treatment is unsuccessful. The symptoms are bladder problems, stiff back, constipation and certain asthma attacks.

Geopathic stress is also characterised by fatigue and a weakening of the immune system, an old disease can reappear or a weakness evolve into a more severe problem.

Young children are very sensitive and they might be affected by nightmares, bed wetting and fatigue.

If these symptoms disappear when one moves to a different location, goes on holiday or sleeps in a different bed, it is wise to study and analyse the quality of the house.

Orientation and cardinal points

Every traditional culture has assigned special meanings to the six directions, North, South, East, West, upwards and downwards. Each direction had its own guardian spirit, its own characteristic and its own purpose.

In ancient Egypt, East and North were positive directions. They were assigned the colour purple, the Spring season, sunrise and draught. West and South were thought of as negative, red and white were their colours, autumn was the corresponding season and these directions were connected to sunset and humidity.

The Chinese have known the property of magnetism for thousands of years. Their first magnetic compasses were used for Feng Shui, the art of geomancy used to define the best sites to erect houses or dig graves. Feng Shui defines eight directions, each with its own characteristics.

North	Black	Wisdom	Career
North-East			Personal growth
East	Green	Goodness	Family Health
South East			Wealth Fortune
South	Red	Spirit	Social standing
South West			Marriage
West	White	Equality	Children
North West			Travel Action

Traditional diagram of Cardinal Directions and Elements (Heliocentric system based on the Northern Hemisphere)

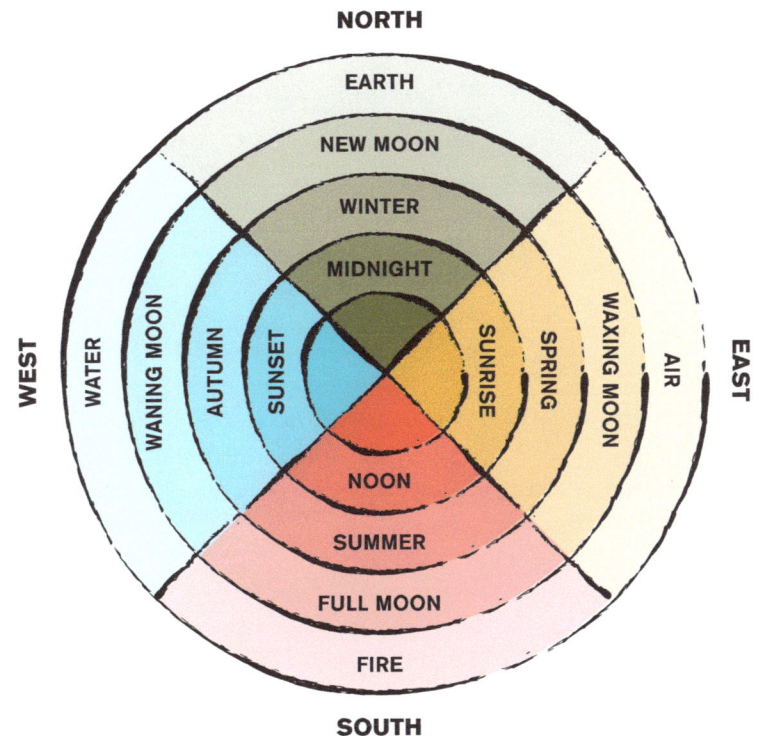

24

Feng Shui gives particular importance to magnetic North which is the recommended orientation of graves and altars dedicated to the ancestors.

In Mali -Africa- the Dogon people always place their bed so as to have their head pointing north. According to Alfred Lambert and Pierre Creuze [7] North has a calming effect, South causes excitement and impatience, East gives joy and West melancholy. Lying with one's head towards North helps to sleep peacefully.

Each direction is influencing our organism differently, activity is stimulated by the East and West directions, rest is enhanced by the North direction.

The importance of correct direction is also known to gardeners. For example, saplings are replanted pointing to the original direction of growth to insure a healthy regrowth. When a Japanese master gardener uses stones in a composition, he will place them exactly the same way he found them in nature so as to respect and be in harmony with the energy flow.

What seems to have been so obvious in many traditions is now being brought to our knowledge by scientific research.

It is thought that bees have such a remarkable sense of direction because their abdomen contains minute particles of magnetite. This material is made of iron and oxygen, it is able to magnetise itself is sensitive to surrounding electromagnetic fields, and it functions as a perfect biological compass. In tests conducted at the University of Hawaii, the bees were able to find food connected to a magnetic field, without seeing the sun, which they also use to orientate themselves.

They were conditioned to find food in a specific area marked by a strong magnet. A strong magnetic field could even attract the bees to brine which they hate. When bees were also equipped with a tiny magnet fixed on their abdomen to disrupt the variations of the magnetic field, they were unable to localise the source of food.

Studies on migratory animals, especially birds, have revealed that they are extremely sensitive to the subtle changes of the geomagnetic field. These birds have minute particles of iron material in their neck muscles. These receptors could be sensitive to changes in the Earth's magnetic field. This ability can be strongly impaired when the magnetic field is under strong disturbance such as high-power lines, power plants, microwaves transmitters... etc.

According to Professor Yves Rocard [8] human beings also possess receptors enabling them to feel the subtle changes of the geomagnetic field. These receptors would be more sensitive and developed in people such as healers and dowsers. These receptors are found in six different areas of the body -two behind the superciliary arches, two in the neck, one in each elbow, two in the lower back, one behind each knee and one under each foot. The body seems more relaxed and comfortable when lying in alignment with the geomagnetic field's natural flow.

In certain cases, there can be strong natural disturbance of the magnetic field, If, for example, there is a major river nearby with a strong current, then it is then preferable to lay with one's head pointing towards the source of the river.

7 A. Lambert- P. Creuze (Etudes sur les influences cosmiques) Maison de la radiesthésie

8 Y. Rocard (Le signal du sourcier) Du

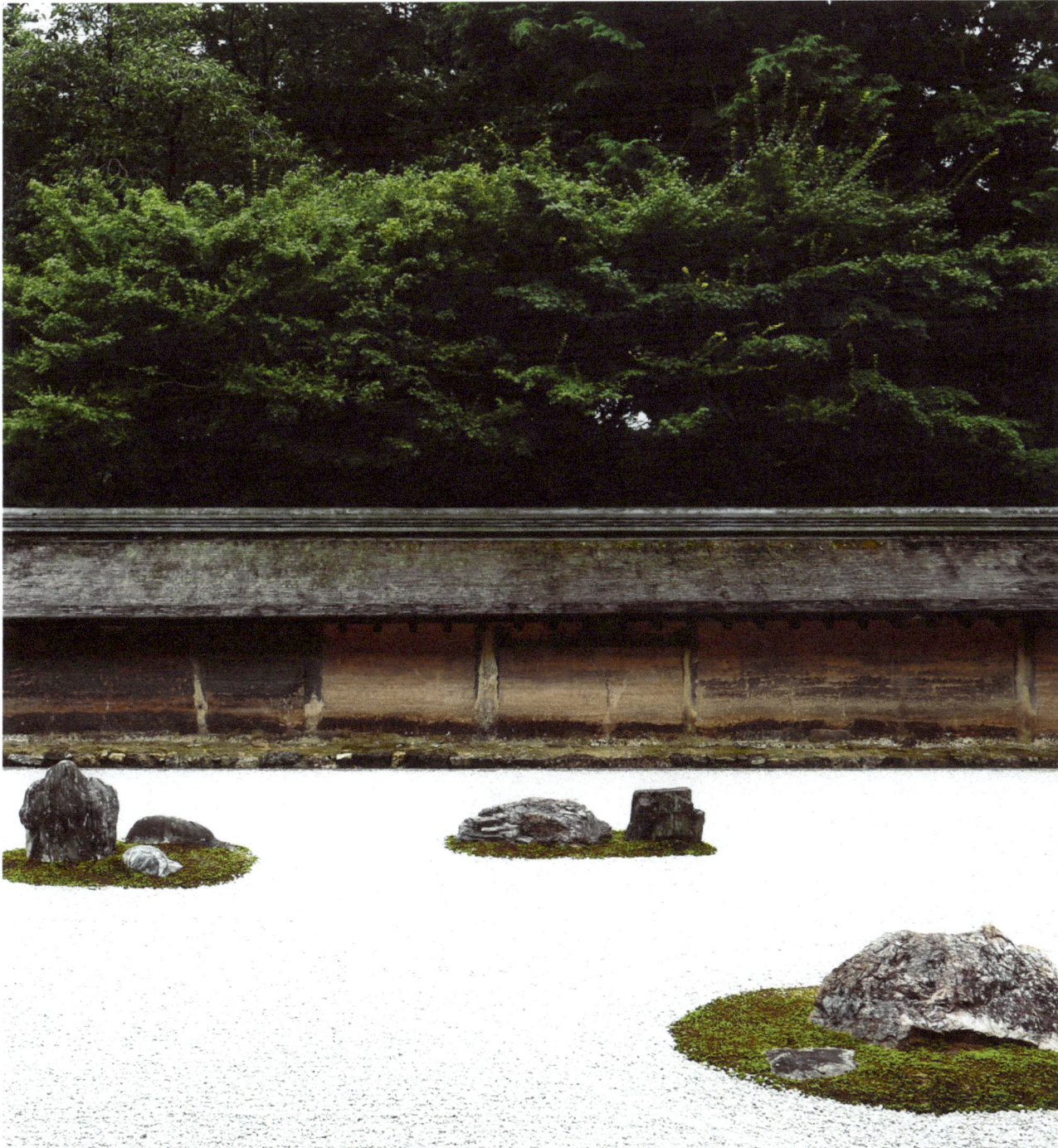

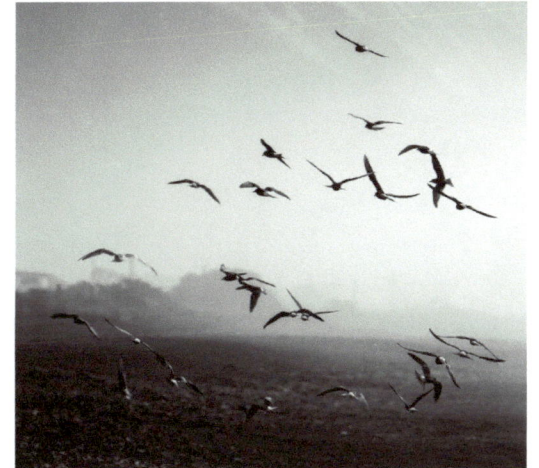

03 /
The Tradition

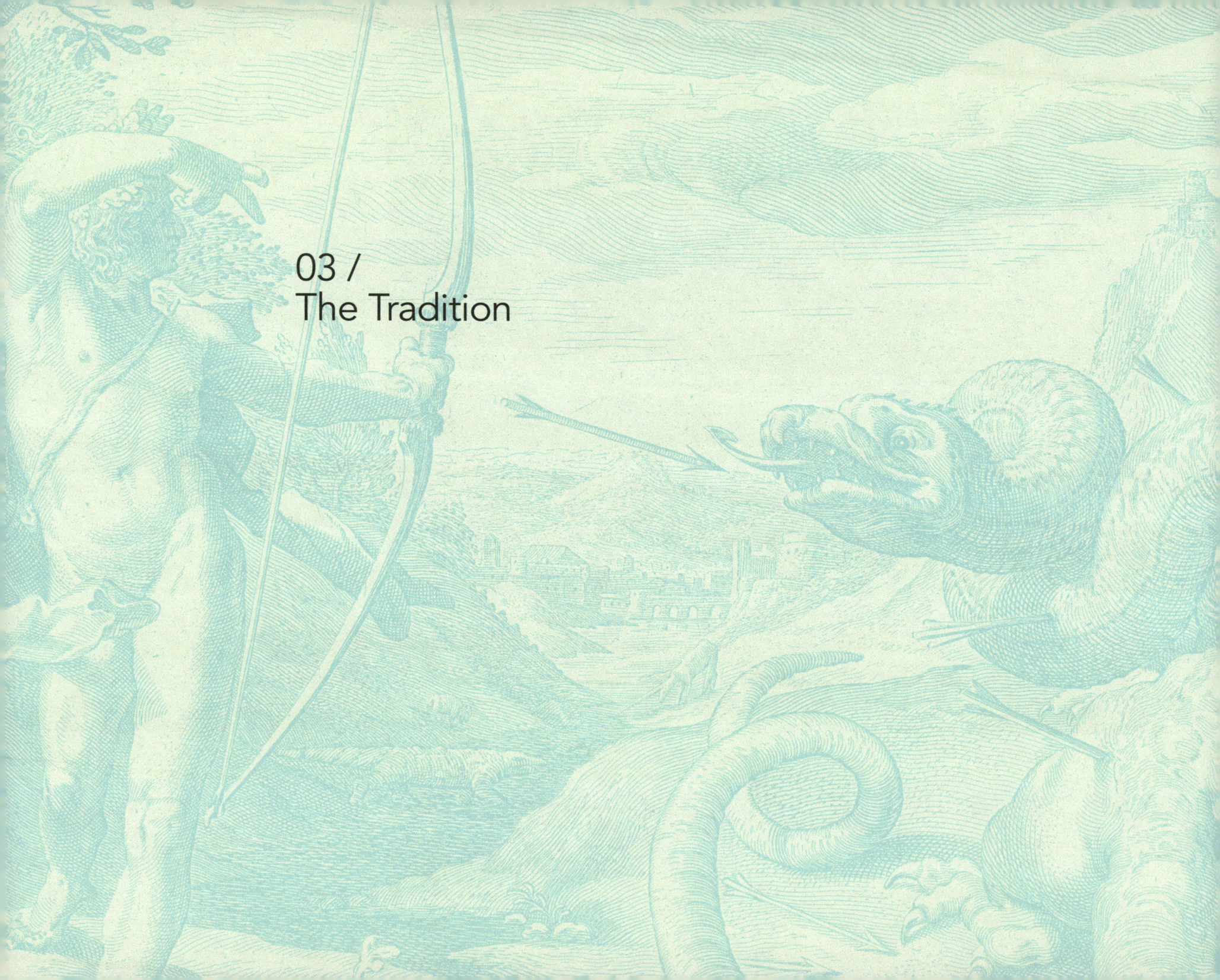

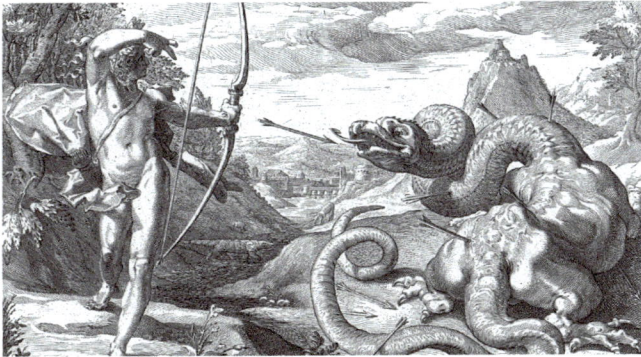

Axis mundi

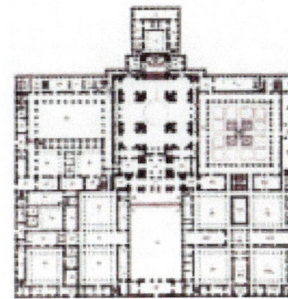

Escurial palace

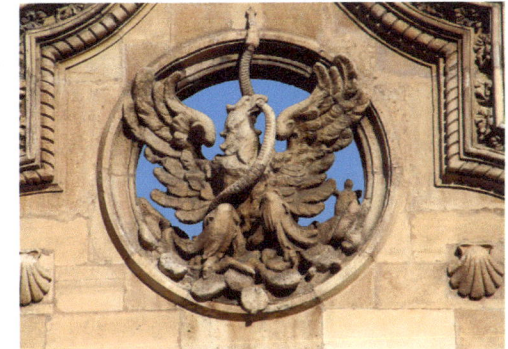

Mexico City Coat of Arms

Since the earliest time in history, a wide set of parameters and rituals have determined suitable building sites. In China, it was defined by Feng Shui, the art of reading the landscape and its influence on a given area. Mountains, lakes rivers and forests were all charged with quantities of energy or Chi, according to their shape, size, and disposition. The relationship between these different elements affected and defined the suitability of sites for particular uses.

Throughout history the foundation of a city or a public building was an occasion of special rituals and dedication to gods, planets or saints. The symbolic aspects of the consecration were most important. An official laying the first stone of an edifice is the remnant of this tradition. The exact moment when the first stone of Cairo was laid corresponded with the ascension

of the planet Mars (El Kaher in Arabic, The Victor). The astrological theme which defines the cosmic affinities of each individual was applied to architecture, the moment of birth of a construction corresponded to laying the first stone.

The start of work on the Escurial Palace, the seat of the Spanish government, was defined by the entrance of the Sun and the Moon in Aries, which presides symbol of high political and military ambition. Furthermore, the building was dedicated to St Lawrence -martyr tortured on a grill- and its plan assumes the shape of a grill. The orientation of an edifice, its position in relation to the stars, the planets, the Sun and the obscure tellurian forces, recognised the hopes for its higher aspirations, what the ancients called the Pillar of the World or "axis mundi".

It was often symbolically illustrated with the image of an archangel representing the cosmic or positive light forces striking a dragon -the tellurian or negative dark forces- or as Apollo slaying the serpent Python. The Abbey of Le Mont St Michel in Normandy, France, is positioned on an axis 64 degrees off North. This direction faces towards the sunrise of the May 8, traditionally the St Michel day of spring. The opposite direction encounters the Sun on the 6th of August, the transfiguration of Christ.

Legend has it that the city of Mexico was built on the site where an eagle was seen devouring a snake, another example of the interaction between cosmic and tellurian forces.

04 /
Topography and environment

29

Every element, Fire, Air, Water and Earth participates in the constant change and evolution of the planet. And today man has earned a place in this combat of giants; his influence can be felt in the very depth of the planet where he is testing nuclear devices, and in the highest levels of the atmosphere where his industrial activities are affecting the climate.

WESTERN TRADITION

The spirit of the place

To the Celts and to the ancient world generally, the land itself was a sacred entity. There was no separation between religion and living. Just like the Aborigines, most cultures realised their origin and dependence on the land.

Each Roman house had its little devotional altar. On it were statues of gods, ancestors and also statues of the "lares" the protector of the household, the "genius loci" or spirit of the place. The Christians considered the genius loci as minor forces which later became the fairies of romantic literature bearing no resemblance to the fayries of the Celtic tradition.

Tellurian forces

The concept of tellurian forces or tellurism is difficult to comprehend depending on whether the source of information comes from science or tradition. From a scientific point of view the tellurian forces are seen as electromagnetic radiation generated and running through the ground according to the degree of humidity and the geological nature of the site. They are considered to have an influence on the human and animal psyche and to be the origin of disturbances affecting telephonic, telegraphic and radio communications.

Though many of the effects of tellurian forces are being studied, the nature of their essence is still unclear.

If we turn to tradition we can find in every culture, independently of its development, references to tellurian forces, in the form of myths, legends and rituals.

For the Celts, it was the Nwywre, the spirit of the depths usually pictured as a serpent, often with a ram's head or as a salamander. The builders of the Druid tradition took great care to locate the path of the Nwywre before erecting stone circles.

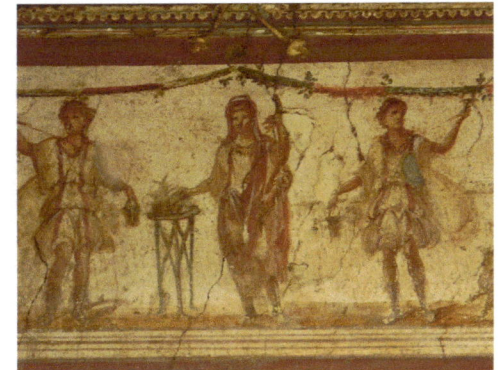

Lares and Genius (Fragment of fresco– Pompeii)

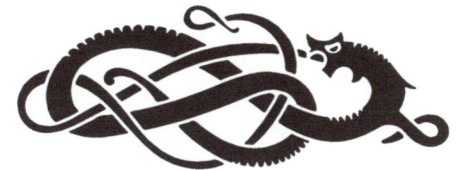

Celtic 'Serpent of Life' - Nwywre or Nyu

30

9 Jean-Louis Bernard (Les Archives de l'Insolite) Éditions du Dauphin

In the Norse mythology, we find Nidhoggr the Earth serpent. For the Chinese it is the dragon, living under the Earth. Its blood, the chi energy, circulates in a mesh of arteries and veins.

For the Aztecs, it was Quetzalcoatl the great snake. For Australian Aborigines, it is the Waggle, the great rainbow serpent which shaped the topography of the continent.

In Greek mythology, the three Cyclops Arges, Brontes and Steropes work ceaselessly in the workshop of Hephaestus under the volcano Etna, like an enormous dynamo generating the planet's energy.

Temples or places of worship and pilgrimage were situated on powerful sources of beneficial tellurism, but it was not for daily use, too much of a good thing can be detrimental to our health. Some areas were systematically avoided because the "breath of the Earth was poisoned". And between these extremes we find a wide range of areas suited to beings attracted to them through resonance.

According to Jean-Louis Bernard (Les Archives de l'Insolite)[9] tellurism can be defined as follows:

- The tellurism has healing power; many temples were places of healing. This tellurian force seems to have been used to heal and purify physical bodies and to digest the dark and rotten emanations of the human psyche.

- It sustains life and plays a significant role in the development of blood and sap. Plants thrive on it and digest it before humans and animals can use it.

- Snakes act as transformers of this energy which they absorb and digest. Through certain rites initiates would absorb it through osmosis.

- Ceremonies and dances around menhirs (Megalithic stone monuments) were the occasion to transfer the energy that had accumulated towards human beings; those who could not digest it would become hysterical. The participants had to be prepared for the rising of this force circulating from the feet up the spine to stop behind the forehead.

- An "overdose" of this energy would cause deformities in the body, particularly the feet, hips and back, as tellurism affect the bone structure.

- The flow of this energy could stimulate certain glands and the production of hormones.

For Aborigines, ants bring this energy up from underground, and in areas where the ants are very active energy can build up and induce fatigue and headaches.

These forces are weaving their paths throughout the landscape and often coincide with migration and pilgrimage routes, punctuated by megaliths, churches and monasteries.

In Australia, they are the "Dream Tracks" or "Song Lines" going from one sacred site to the other.

As we encounter these tellurian forces, we should define their qualities and, analyse and know them as they emerge at the site. The quality of a location is expressed by the fantasy of nature. The interplay of different elements creates different environments which in turn moulds the characteristics of the inhabitants.

They are the energies of the four elements, fire, water, air and earth and their interplay. They are all present, but one usually dominates.

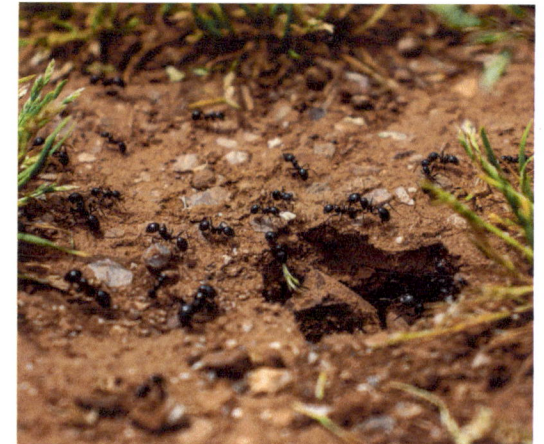

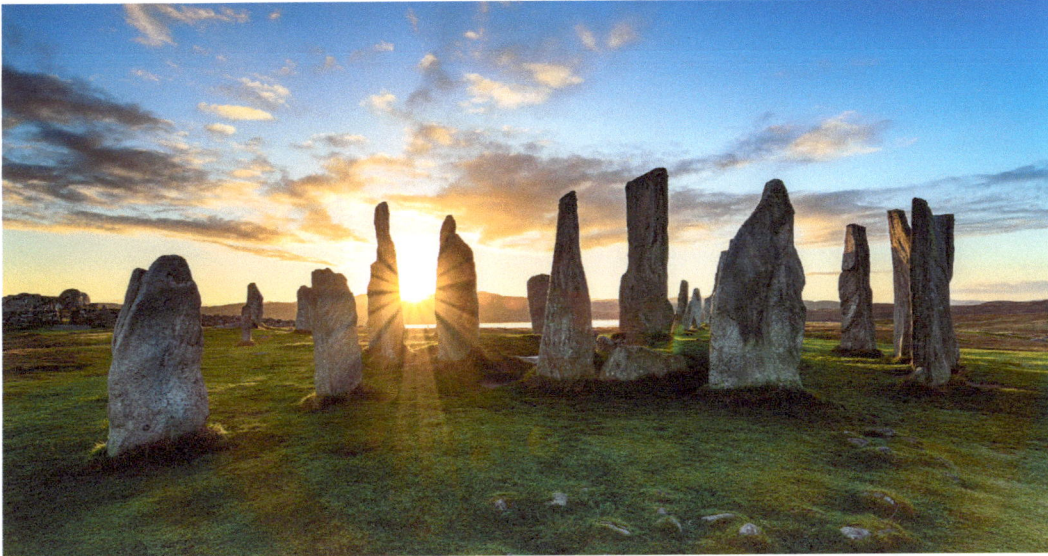

Fire: (hot and dry)

The fire element reveals itself in warm and dry regions, in sulphurous soil, iron mines and volcanic areas. It is a symbol of purification. Known to cure certain skin problems sulphurous springs were sought after since antiquity.

Water: (cold and humid)

Every human settlement has developed in the vicinity of water. In addition, as a prerequisite for survival, it has become a symbol of the gift of life. Even though technology has enabled us to transport water far from its source, the presence of water on a given site is a great asset and can dramatically modify the quality of the environment. Water will improve a site when running fresh from a deep well, a spring, a running creek or it might render the site inhospitable when lying stagnant and rotting whether above or below ground. Vast expenses of water such as lakes and seas have a calming effect. Underground water stream can stimulate life energies though this can be detrimental to certain individuals.

Air: (hot and humid)

The air energy resides in elevated places and in wooded areas, trees being mediators between the winds and the earth. The Oak was dedicated to Zeus, god of thunder, often attracts lightning because this tree tends to grow along tellurian lines.

The nymph Daphne, daughter of the river god Peneus, refused the advances of Apollo and was thus changed into a laurel tree. This tree is known to protect houses because it does not grow above underground water streams.

The cypress tree is associated with Cronus, the Greek god of time, and represents immortality; it is often planted in cemeteries and thrives in dry areas.

Air energy stimulates the psyche and the thinking process but it can also excite the nervous system and provoke restlessness. Exposed areas should be protected from an excess of wind by planting trees.

Earth: (cold and dry)

Earth energy is particularly dominant in areas where the key features are caves and mountains. These energies have always been held in awe by mankind. Rocks, hills, mountains and caverns have all been used as object or places of worship. Megaliths were used to indicate where the tellurian forces were particularly active. The quality of earth energy is to calm and to ground the psyche.

32

The geomagnetic grid

When considering a homogenous geological site, the energy on the surface is not distributed evenly or randomly. As metal dust will gather according to the flowing patterns of a magnetic field generated in a metal plate -Cymatics, the energy will radiate in a pattern of lines, crossing and neutral zones.

The density of the radiation will be stronger in the lines and even more so on the crossing of these lines.

The observation of these grids has confirmed that they cover the entire surface of the planet and become tighter towards the poles.

The Peyre grid:

In France Dr Francois Peyre, a pioneer in this field, studied the presence of a geomagnetic grid oriented North-South, its dimension being between seven and eight metres.

The Hartmann grid:

In Germany Dr Ernst Hartmann (Director of the Research Committee for Geobiology, Eberbach- Waldkatzenbach- Waldbrunn) of Heidelberg University is a pioneer in Cosmo-tellurian radiation research and is considered to be the father of geobiology. He is the first to have used this term in the 1930s. He established the existence of what is now known as the Hartmann grid, or H grid. It is a global grid oriented north-south.

Its lines, or walls, are 21 cm wide and run from pole to pole. In the temperate latitudes, the space between these lines is 2.5 m in the east-west direction and 2 m in the north-south direction. The grid is thus composed of ener-getically neutral areas between the walls, which are defined as low radiation areas and the high radiation areas at the points where the walls cross.

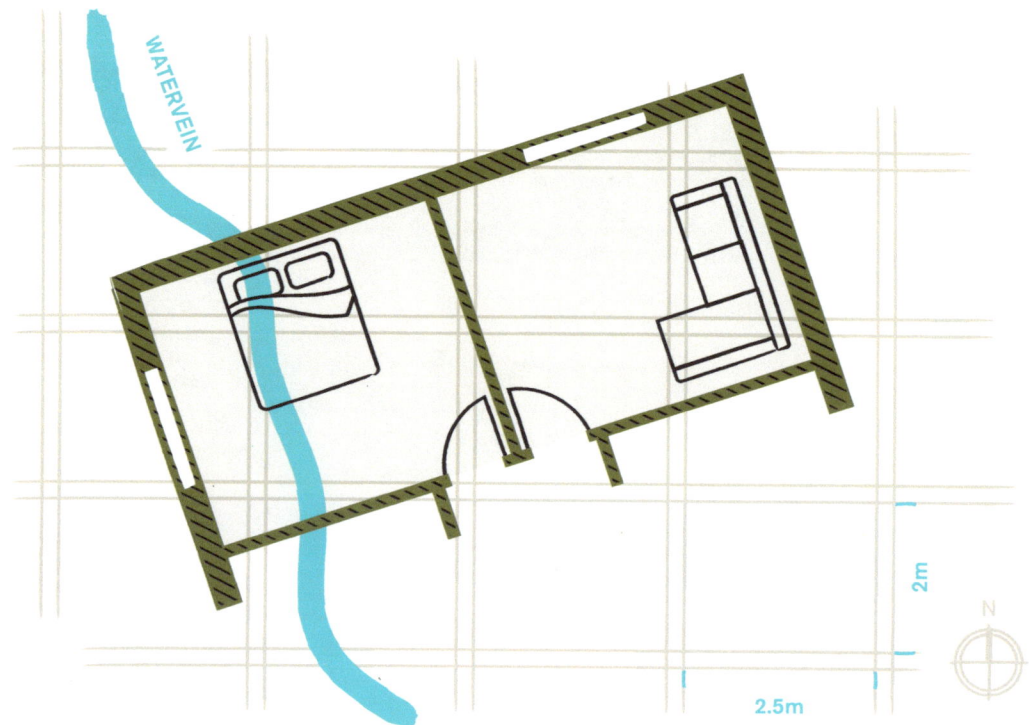

The Hartmann grid

33

10 Le rayonnement de la terre et son influence sur la vie (R. Endros) Ed. Le Signal

The crossing points of these lines are considered to be unhealthy if one is to remain over them for extended periods, as in a bed or at a workstation for example. The regularity of the H grid can be affected by the nature of the ground, geological faults, and underground water streams as well as man-made disturbances such as high-tension power lines, roads and railroads along which the H grid is permanently tighter and contracted.

The effect of a crossing, or knot, in the H grid can be amplified by local geological characteristics such as faults and water veins making this area potentially dangerous.

According to Professor Robert Endros, author of *"The earth radiation and its influence on Life"*[10] trees growing on the crossings of the grid are prone to be struck by lightning, especially when near or above an underground stream. Most trees or plants showing deformities and abnormalities are found on knots of the H grid. On these the Romans used to build sham wells dedicated to Jupiter and consecrated to fulgur conditum, or buried lightning.

Animals and young children have not lost their instinct to feel if a place is healthy or not. In the morning children can often be seen oriented differently from when they were tucked in. It is wise to see if the bed is well positioned. Sensitive adults will not sit in a particular spot often without being able to explain why they feel uncomfortable. Animals in pastures will avoid a disturbed zone which is obvious by looking at the area that has been left un-grazed.

Engraving in the "Speculum metallurgicum politissimum" (18th century) showing prospectors using a divining rod.

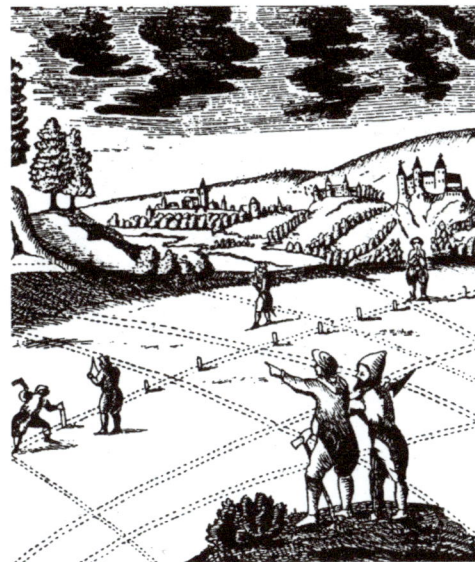

FENG-SHUI

DEFINITION

There is not in the Western tradition a system as well structured as Feng Shui to read and interpret a site. A Feng Shui site reading gives another level of comprehension; it includes the intricate web of relationships between man, the future use of the site and the topography. Feng Shui offers guidelines for the good positioning of a building on a site.

Feng-Shui literally means wind and water and has often been incorrectly translated as geomancy. It is a popular geography and medicine which has been in use in China for thousands of years.

As geography, it is the art of designing dwellings for the living and the dead to be in harmony with the local flow of energy, or chi.

It is the harmonious balance between the female principle, yin and the male principle, yang, the five elements, the six energies and the ever-present breath of chi pervading all nature through the study of topography, site morphology, climate and vegetation.

As a medicine, it is meant as a protection against diseases before they manifest. It is based on the same principles as Chinese medicine which strives to maintain and stimulate the life-giving

34

flow of chi. Both Feng- Shui and acupuncture use a similar terminology, in Feng- Shui "Long-Mai" designates the "Dragon's veins" which channel the Earth's energy and "Lao-mai" designates the meridians distributing the chi energy throughout the human body. The term "Shuey" refers to both a point of acupuncture and a favourable site.

Feng-Shui is also used for town planning, architecture, landscaping and decorating. It integrates optimally the human structures on the site by defining their orientation, shape, colours and proportions.

PHILOSOPHY

Taoism is the framework for an integrated system embracing every aspect of traditional Chinese life. Town planning, architecture, art, music, poetry, medicine and even cooking are all based on this mystical doctrine promoting union with nature.

It is helpful to have some knowledge of Taoism to be able to understand the principles on which lies the traditional Chinese view of the world. The Daodejing or Tao Te King, The Sacred Book of Tao was written around 300 BC by Lao Tzu.

It explains that at the beginning was the void, the unnameable, the unknowable out of which came the One, The Tao, the primordial cause of all existence. In its first movement, its first breath, it created the male principle, Yang.

When the action reached its limits, there was a rest out of which was born Yin, the female principle. The alternate movements of action and rest, the first polarity gave birth in their perpetual transformation to all creation and all living beings including humans. The vital energy bringing to life both principles is called Chi.

The theory of Yin and Yang is a fundamental concept and pervades Chinese thinking it is also its most popular aspect known in the West.

The Tai Chi is the graphic symbol used to depict the concept of Yin and Yang in a state of equilibrium, it is however the symbol of a dynamic in constant motion and mutation. The white area represents Yang and the black area Yin. The Tai Chi is the expression of the whole; both Yin and Yang are intimately intertwined to show that nothing is entirely Yin or entirely Yang. Even in the greatest manifestation of an energy type we can see the seed of the other, depicted by both a white dot in the black area and a black dot in the white one.

In the Suwen, the second part of a treaty of Acupuncture called Neijing, written at the beginning of the Christian era the concept of Yin and Yang is explained in the following manner.

"There is Yang inside Yin and Yin inside Yang. From dawn to noon heavenly Yang is Yang inside Yang. From noon to twilight heavenly

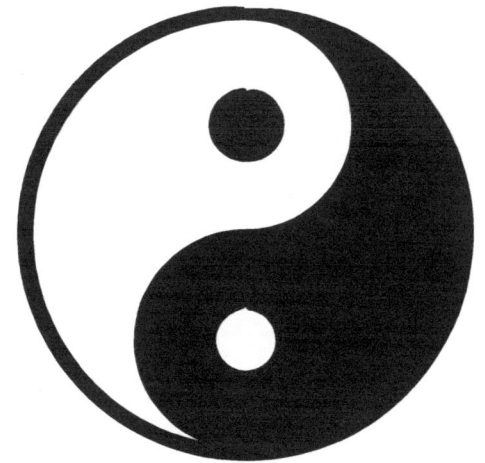

Tai chi

Yang is Yin inside Yang. From sundown to midnight heavenly Yin is Yin inside Yin and from midnight to sunrise Yin is Yang inside Yin."

GREAT YANG   **LITTLE YANG**   **LITTLE YIN**   **GREAT YIN**

YANG

HEAVEN

LAKE   **WIND**

N

NE   **NW**

FIRE   **WATER**

E   **W**

SE   **SW**

S

THUNDER   **MOUNTAIN**

EARTH

YIN

PAKUA

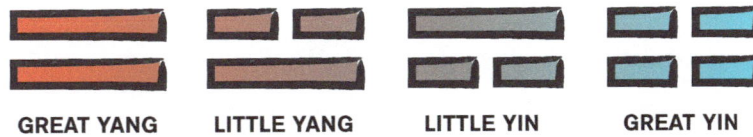

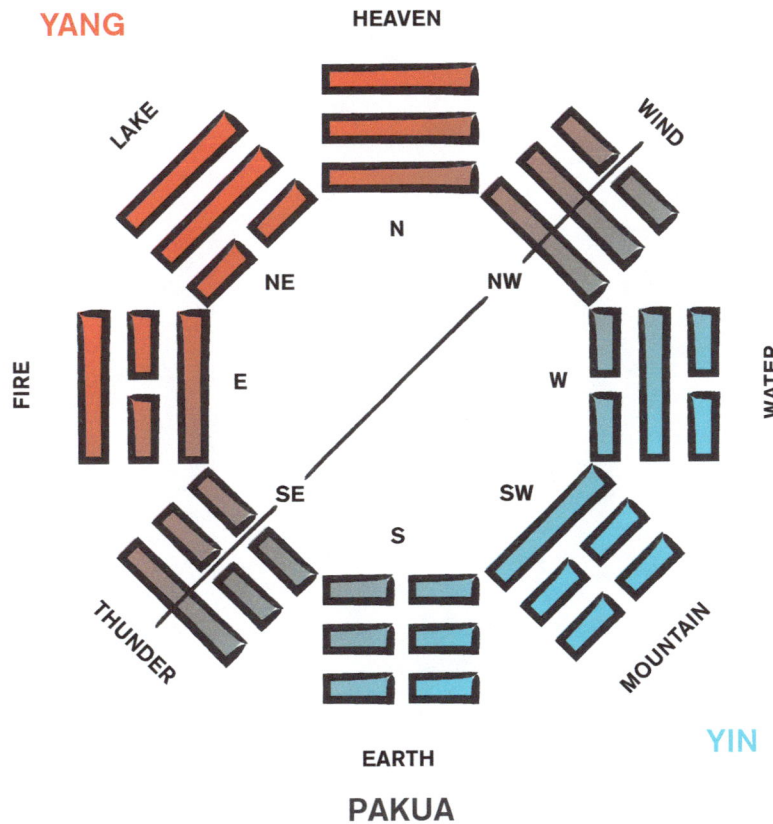

According to Taoism, Man is the association of the energies of the Cosmos (Yang) with the energies of the Earth (Yin); He transmutes these energies for the benefit of His evolution thanks to the four seasons (time).

Yang: The male principle is manifested in action, expansion, light, heat, heaven, etc.

Yin: The female principle manifests itself in rest, contraction, darkness, cold, earth, etc.

Yin and yang can also be understood as a simple binary system in which yang is expressed by a continuous line (—) and yin by a broken line (- -). The combination of these two lines indicates the four main stages of yin and yang

If a third line is added we obtain the set of eight Trigrams (Pakua) which was revealed to the legendary Emperor Fu Hsi by a dragon coming out of the Yellow River.

When multiplying this set by itself we obtain the sixty-four hexagrams of the I Ching, representing all the transformation cycles through the unceasing mutation of Yin and Yang.

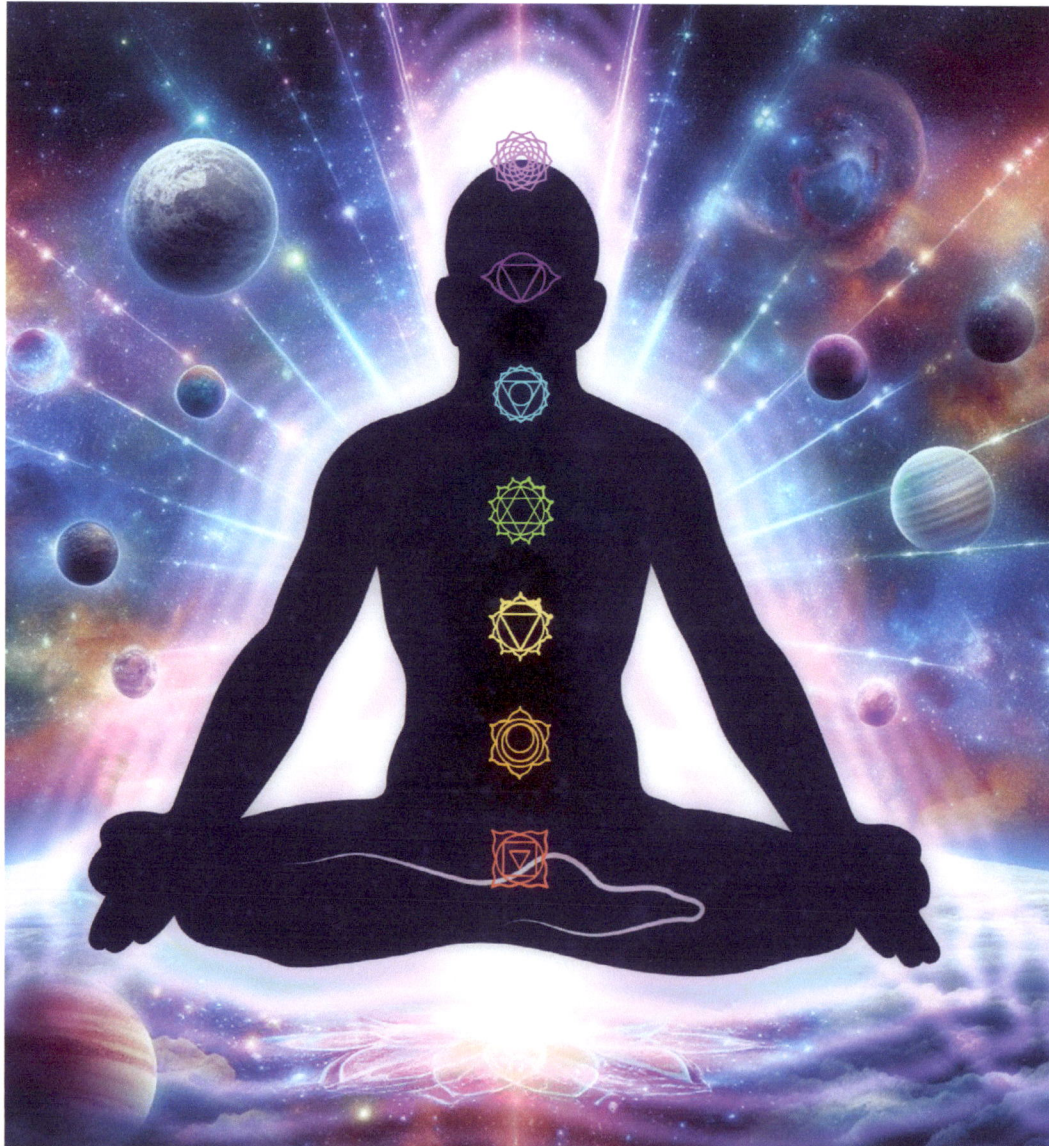

THE CHI ENERGY, THE COSMIC BREATH

Chi is the natural force which permeates the entire universe. According to traditional Chinese medicine it is a subtle energy in constant movement. This movement is literally the activity of life as well as one of the constituents of our body.

Chi is also called "the blood of the dragon", circulating in the terrestrial body through a network of channels as it does also through the meridians of the human body.

It is the ki of Japan. In the Hindu tradition, it is called prana and in ancient Greece, pneuma.

The quality of a site depends on the quantity and on the quality of chi. It should not be stagnant and should not escape the site too quickly. When the energy is not renewed regularly it becomes diseased and an overexposed site is easily depleted of life energy.

37

The five elements follow each other in the seasonal order. In this natural order, each element generates the next, it was traditionally called the Mother- Son order. In this harmonious order, the chi energy can circulate with the most beneficial effect.

THE FIVE ELEMENTS

The Chinese emperor was the link between heaven and earth, the prosperity of his people depended on his rigorous compliance to the laws ruling each of his actions, down to the clothes he wore and the food he ate. These laws were dictated by the expression of the five elements which regulates the quality of all mutations in space and in time. In space, each element rules a direction and in time each element rules a year, a season and an hour. Furthermore, each element rules a category of living entities or objects.

In the Chinese system, the element Metal corresponds to the West and Autumn, the element Water corresponds to the North and Winter, Wood corresponds to the Eastern direction and Spring and Fire is related to South and Summer. As for the element Earth, it relates to the Centre and the End of Summer (1), it is the mediator between all the other elements, it is also related to the last eighteen days of each season. In the Southern Hemisphere, north and south should be inversed as the Northern direction relates to the equator and the summer sun.

Based on this system elaborate tables of correspondence were set to classify almost everything into five categories ruled by one of these elements.

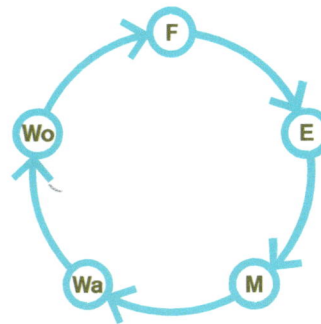

1) Mother/Son generation

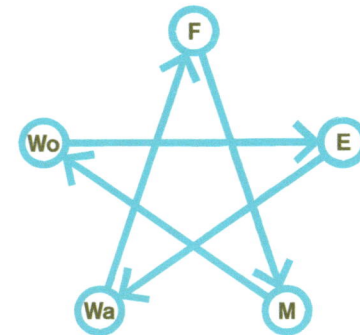

2) Mother /Grandson destruction

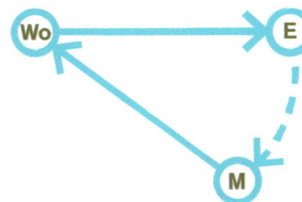

3) Controlling principle

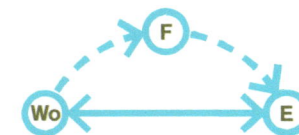

4) Correcting principle

38

When the Mother element destroys its "Grandson" (2), bypassing the element that usually follows, we then have the cycle of destruction and the chi becomes impure. Both cycles are supposed to function simultaneously as the inhale and the exhale of nature.

A balance between the elements is created by the principles of control and correction.

With the controlling principle (3), the wood element for example is too strong and "dries" the earth but since the earth generates metal the latter helps the earth by cutting the wood, the earth thus regains its humidity and harmony.

In the example of the correcting principle (4) we see that when the element wood is over abundant and disrupts the earth the fire element acts as a correcting factor. The wood feeds the fire which in turn feeds the earth with its ashes which then feeds the wood. The whole process is harmonised.

These principles are used throughout Chinese arts and sciences.

Throughout the year, the Chinese emperor had to move in the five different wings of his palace according to the seasons. During spring, he resided in the east wing and, in summer he lived in the south wing called the Luminous Palace. At the end of summer he moved to the centre of the palace, the Supreme Hall, in autumn the

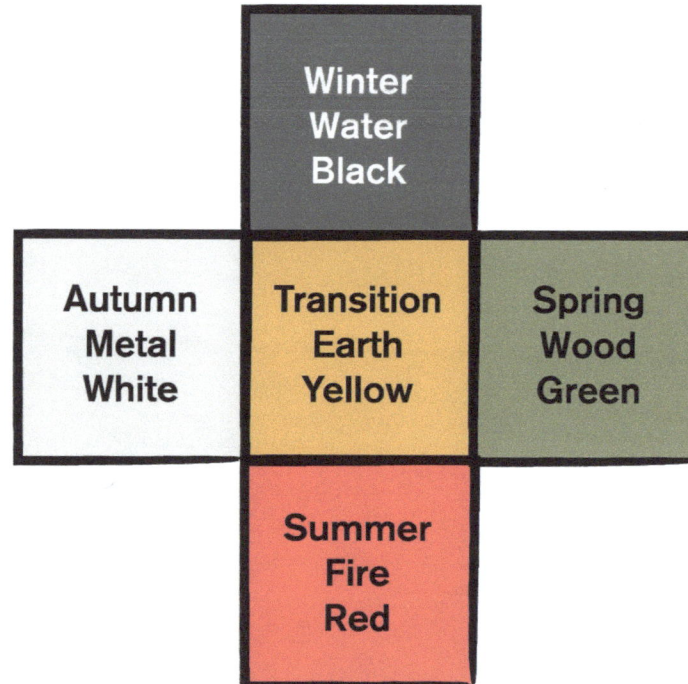

	Winter Water Black	
Autumn Metal White	Transition Earth Yellow	Spring Wood Green
	Summer Fire Red	

Ming Tang (Bright Palace)

west wing was his residence, the Hall of beauty. Finally, in winter the emperor ended the yearly cycle in the Mystery Hall, in the north wing.

39

House built in Hamilton Hill (Western Australia) in 2006 using the Ming Tang (Bright Palace) layout principles. The local climate is defined as yang, hot and dry Mediterranean.

The Red Dragon (fire element) faces the sun (north in the Southern Hemisphere) and the Black Turtle (water element) faces South, it includes the bathroom, laundry and circulation space.

The walls are made of rammed earth (yin) to correct the excess of yang energy.

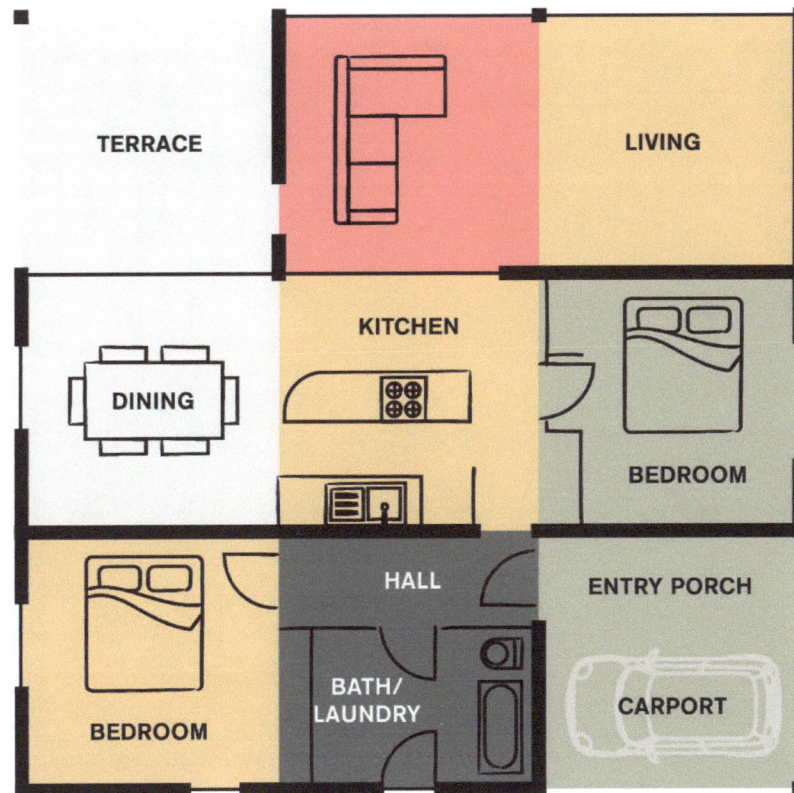

TERRACE

LIVING

KITCHEN

DINING

BEDROOM

HALL

ENTRY PORCH

BEDROOM

BATH/ LAUNDRY

CARPORT

N

SEASONAL HIERARCHY OF ELEMENTS

MODES	POWERFUL	ENERGETIC	WEAK	MODERATING	INACTIVE
SEASONS					
SPRING	WOOD	FIRE	EARTH	METAL	WATER
SUMMER	FIRE	EARTH	METAL	WATER	WOOD
END OF SUMMER	EARTH	METAL	WATER	WOOD	FIRE
AUTUMN	METAL	WATER	WOOD	FIRE	EARTH
WINTER	WATER	WOOD	FIRE	EARTH	METAL

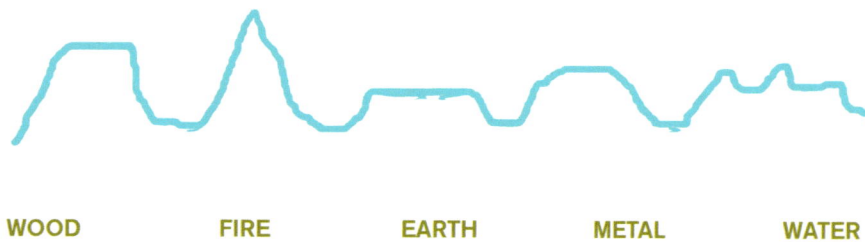

WOOD   FIRE   EARTH   METAL   WATER

Rather than a set of qualities the five elements are more like processes woven in time and space.

According to Feng Shui the topography of a particular area is perceived as a reflection of cosmic forces thus the different shapes of mountains are classified into five categories, each belonging to one of the five elements.

The ideal site is found where the mountains are located in the "Mother-Son" order. This occurs very rarely in nature. It follows that when the mountains are standing in the order of destruction the site is not considered favourable. However, Feng Shui is not a passive system and one is allowed to transform the shape of the scenery to improve the quality of a site.

41

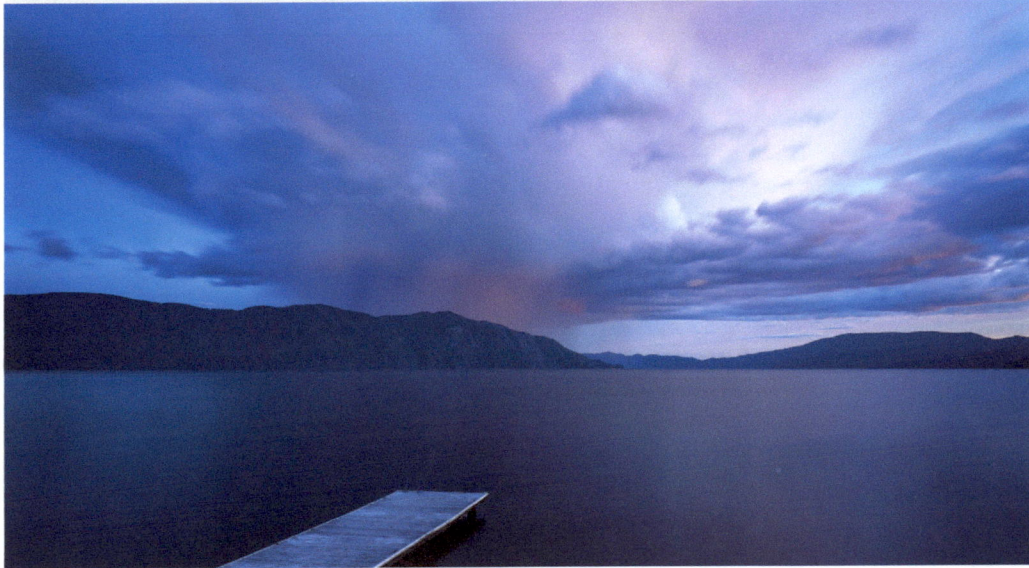

equatorial areas such as the northern part of Australia, Indonesia, Africa and South America.

The Yin climates:

- **Hyper yin** climates are found in the North and the South poles and in very high altitude.

- **Yin** climates are found in the temperate zone in mountainous areas such as the Alps, Himalayas, Rocky Mountains and the Andes.

- **Little yin** climates are found in temperate zones and include Central Europe, Canada, the USA, Tasmania and New Zealand.

There are two main types of climates on the planet, yin and yang and they can be subdivided into the following categories.

THE SIX CELESTIAL ENERGIES

Cosmic energy reaches Earth through the spectrum of six stages of yin and yang named the Six Energies. There are three yang energies, hyper yang, yang, little yang and three yin energies, hyper yin, yin and little yin.

In Chinese tradition, the weather is the result of the interaction of the Five Elements and the Six Energies. These complex relationships can be simplified into the following classification.

The yang climates:

- **Hyper yang** climates are found in deserts such as Australia's deserts, the Sahara and the Kalahari in Africa and in the Arabic Peninsula.

- **Yang climates** are found in the sub-tropical areas such as the Middle East, around the Mediterranean Sea, California and the southern part of Australia.

- **Little Yang** climates are characterised by heat and humidity and are found in tropical and

Yang = Hot

Great Yang = Hot and Dry

Little Yang = Hot and Humid

Yin = Cold

Little Yin = Cold and Dry

Great Yin = Cold and Humid

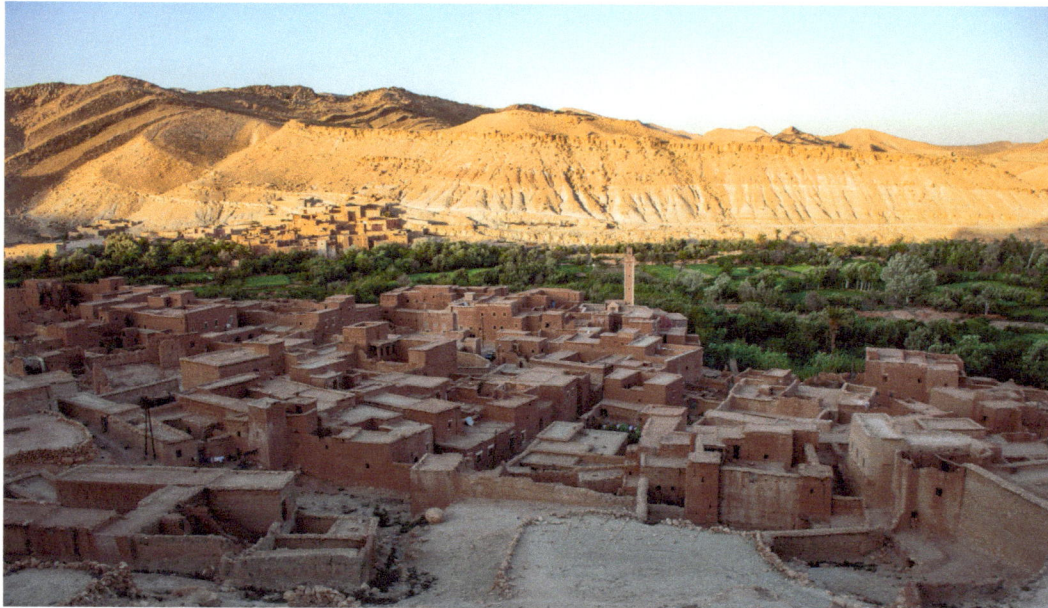

Moroccan Village

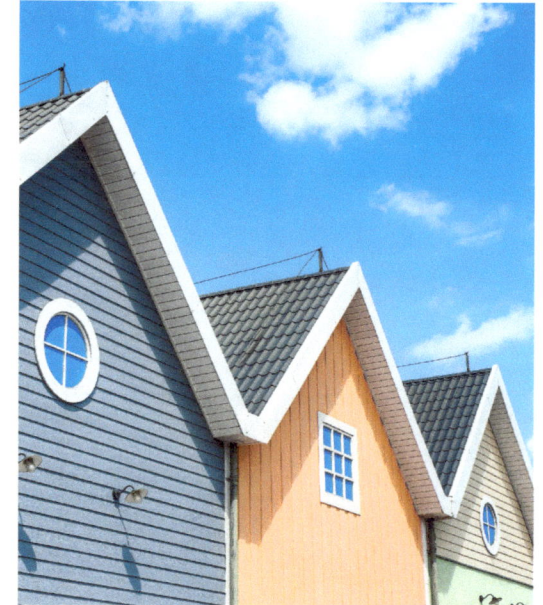

Wooden houses in Sweden

SHAPES IN HARMONY WITH THE LOCAL ENERGY

The shape of a building, its structure and its position will define its ability to absorb a harmonious proportion of yin and yang energies. Depending on the local climate, these parameters can greatly vary. Traditional architecture styles can give us clues as to how local conditions will define the planning of a house and the choice of building materials.

Desert nomads live in tents which are yang structures in a Hyper Yang climate, and the Inuits build yin structures like igloos in a Hyper Yin climate. Under these extreme conditions, we see that the populations are traditionally nomadic, as if the force of a concentrated energy flow was too stressful to allow them to remain too long in one area.

In yang climates of North Africa houses are built to maximise the flow of yin energy. This is achieved by the use of flat rooves to reflect the yang energy from above. Thick rammed earth or brick walls radiate yin energy.

In the yin climates of Northern Europe, we see the yang wooden structures of Swedish houses covered with steep rooves to enable the downward flow of yang energy. We see the same steep roof in some buildings found in equatorial jungles; usually these houses are built on stilts, even though in a yang climate these houses have been conceived to counterbalance the strong yin feeling generated by the very high humidity content of the air.

43

DESIGN WITH THE FIVE ELEMENTS

Once the essence and the quality of each element is understood, as well as its interaction in space and time with the other elements, we can establish a classification of diverse types of building and architectural elements to harmonise the habitat with the climate, the site and the inhabitants.

ELEMENTS	NATURAL SHAPES	BUILT SHAPES	HSIANG
WOOD			
FIRE			
EARTH			
METAL			
WATER			

Geology

The Yin-Yang polarity of an area is determined by the nature of its ground composition.

Yang: Sedimentary rocks

Yin: Metamorphic rocks and igneous rocks

Fire: Limestone, chalk, gypsum

Wood: Sandstone, clay

Earth: Eroded rocks, mixed rocks

Metal: Basalt, granite

Water: Schist, mica, gneiss

Climates

Yang: Hot and dry

Yin: Cold and humid

Fire: Hot and dry, deserts

Wood: Hot and humid, tropical

Earth: Changing, temperate

Metal: Cold and dry, mountains

Water: Cold and humid, polar regions

Topography

The relief of the land will define the polarity of the site.

Yang: Mountainous, concave, uneven

Yin: Gentle forms, valleys

Fire: Peak, cliff, sudden break

Wood: Slope, embankment

Earth: Hills, plateau

Metal: Plain, beach

Water: Swamps, river basin

Dwelling types

Dwellings are designed as a response to a climate.

Yang: To protect against cold and humid weather

Yin: To protect against hot and dry weather

Fire: Wooden buildings with steep rooves

Wood: Chalet, timber frame

Earth: Brick houses

Metal: Vaulted rooves, domes

Water: Flat rooves, underground houses

Living areas

Yang: Spaces generating activities, communication, Working, eating

Yin: Spaces generating rest, sleep, meditation, Storage

Fire: Living room

Wood: Kitchen

Earth: Bathroom, meditation

Metal: Bedroom

Water: Storage, cellar

Roofing materials

Yang: Ventilated roof, material which allows breathing

Yin: Waterproof material

Fire: Thatched roof, vegetal fibre

Wood: Tiles

Earth: Slate

Metal: Metal roof

Water: Bitumen

Structure

Yang: Visible elements

Yin: Invisible elements

Fire: Roof

Wood: Walls

Earth: Openings

Metal: Floors

Water: Foundations

Openings

Yang: Lets light and air through

Yin: protects against rain and intruders

Fire: Oriels

Wood: Bay window

Earth: Door, window

Metal: Fixed window, glass bricks

Water: Shutters, blinds

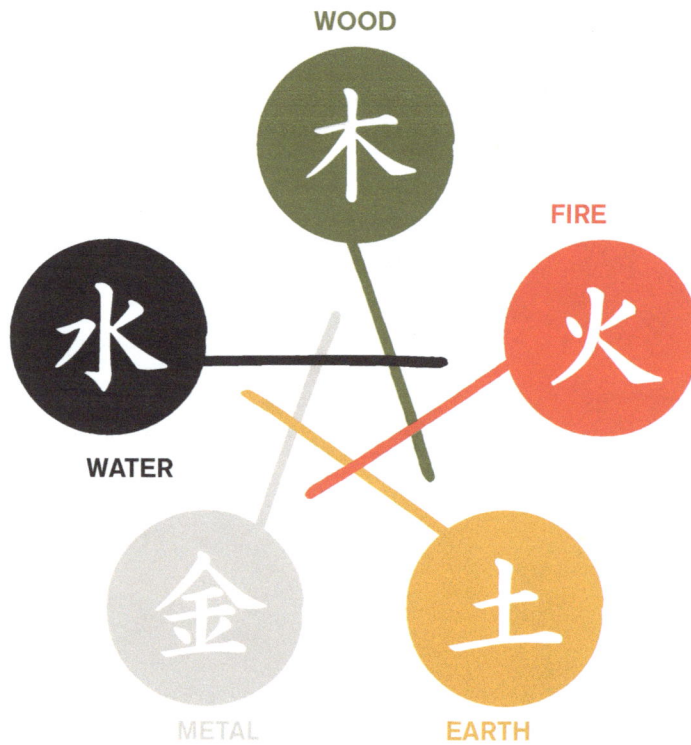

WOOD

木

FIRE

火

水
WATER

金
METAL

土
EARTH

The Chinese system, being holistic, encompasses all aspects of life, from medicine and diet, emotions and psychological traits to music and philosophy, as shown on the non-exhaustive Chinese Symbolic Concordance Table below.

BODY AND PERSONALITY TYPE ACCORDING TO THE FIVE ELEMENTS

	BODY	PERSONALITY
WOOD	thin and lean bodies, broad high forehead	driven with a sense of purpose, can become irritated
FIRE	well proportioned, can have a ruddy complexion	energetic and passionate, can be volatile
EARTH	larger bodies, square face, strong jaw	caring and reliable, have a tendency to worry
METAL	strong and muscular, strong cheekbones	intellectual and organised, can be critical
WATER	round and soft bodies, large eyes	determined and wise, can be fearful and indecisive

CHINESE SYMBOLIC CONCORDANCES TABLE

ELEMENTS	WOOD	FIRE	EARTH	METAL	WATER
DIRECTIONS	EAST	SOUTH	CENTRE	WEST	NORTH
NUMBERS	8 (YOUNG YIN)	7 (YOUNG YANG)	8 (SYNTHESIS)	9 (OLD YANG)	6 (OLD YIN)
COLOURS	GREEN	RED	YELLOW	WHITE	BLACK
PLANETS	JUPITER	MARS	SATURN	VENUS	MERCURY
PALACES	GREEN DRAGON	RED PHOENIX	URSA MAJOR	WHITE TIGER	BLACK TURTLE
SEASONS	SPRING	SUMMER	END OF SEASONS	AUTUMN	WINTER
HOURS	5H-7H	11H-13H	TRANSITIONS	17H-19H	23H-1H
ENERGIES	WIND	FIRE	HUMIDITY	DROUGHT	COLD
CLIMATES	WINDY	HOT	RAINY	DRY	COLD
SYMBOLS	STARS	SUN	EARTH	HOUSES	MOON
PARTS OF HOUSE	DOORS	FIREPLACE	COURTYARD	ENTRANCE DOOR	WELL/PATHS
FOODS	WHEAT	BEANS	WHITE MILLET	OLEAGINOUS SEEDS	YELLOW MILLET
ANIMAL KINDS	WITH SCALES	WITH FEATHERS	WITH BARE SKIN	WITH HAIRS	WITH SHELLS
DOMESTIC ANIM	SHEEP	CHICKEN	CATTLE	DOG	PIG
TREES	THUYA	CATALPA	MAPLE	CHESTNUT	ACACIA
EVOLUTION	BIRTH	GROWTH	TRANSFORMATION	DECLINE	STAGNATION/DEATH
ORGANS	LIVER	HEART	SPLEEN	LUNGS	KIDNEYS
ENTRAILS	GALLBLADDER	SMALL INTESTINE	STOMACH	LARGE INTESTINE	BLADDER
FINGERS	THUMB	MIDDLE	RING	INDEX	LITTLE
SENSE ORGANS	EYES	TONGUE	MOUTH	NOSE/SKIN	EARS
TASTES	SOUR	BITTER	SWEET	PUNGENT	SALTY
SMELLS	RANCID	BURNED	PERFUMED	OF RAW MEAT	ROTTEN
HUMAN ACTIVITY	SIGHT/KNOWLEDGE	SPEECH/ORDERJOY	WILLPOWER/WISDOM	EARING/HARMONY	GESTURE/GOODNESS
EMOTIONS	ANGER	JOY	REFLEXION	GRIEF	FEAR
TISSUES	NERVES/MUSCLES	BLOOD	MUCOUS MEMBRANE	SKIN/HAIR/NAILS	BONES/MARROW
REACTIONS	SWEAT/SCREAM	LAUGHS/FIDGETING	SING/BURP	COUGH/CRY	MOAN/TREMBLE
MOVEMENT	TURN LEFT	GO AHEAD	IMMOBILITY	TURN RIGHT	GO BACKWARDS
VIRTUES	GOODNESS	SPIRITUALITY	FAITH	JUSTICE	WISDOM
SOUNDS	SHOOO	HOOO	WOOD	SHHH	SHUAI
MUSIC NOTES	A	C	F	G	D

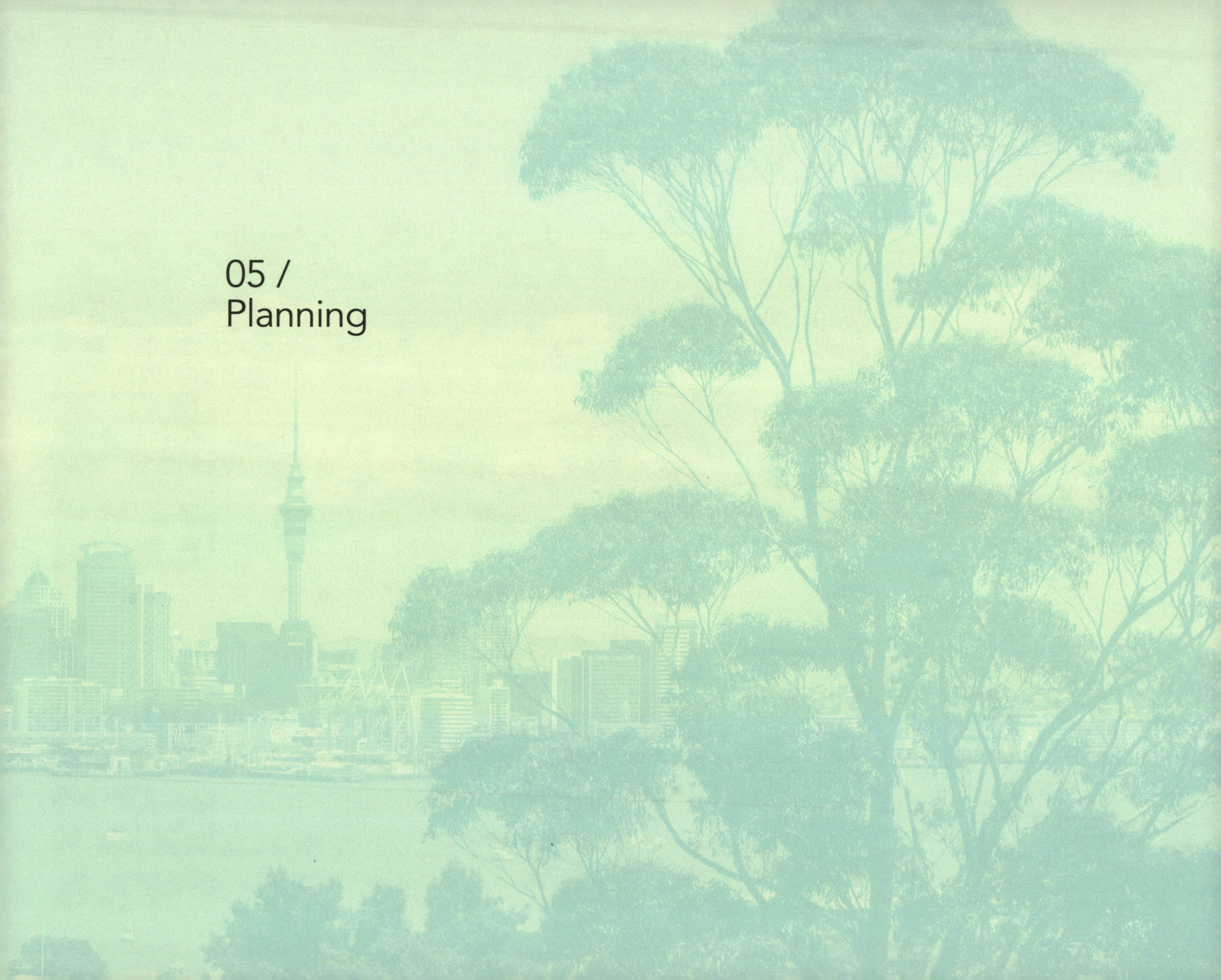

05 /
Planning

49

11 Nigel Pennick
(The Ancient Science
of Geomancy) CRCS
Publications

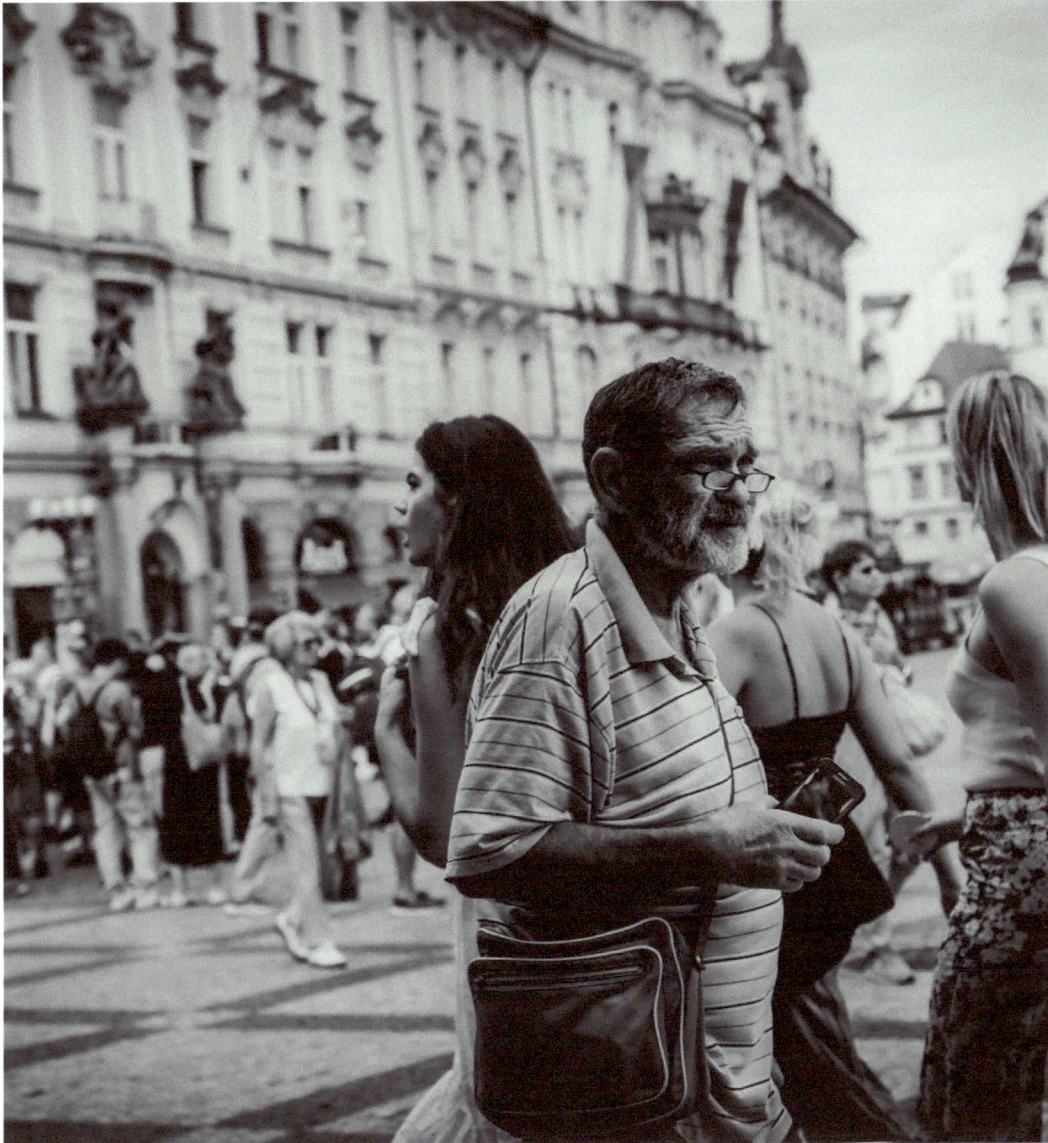

Building a city or a town has always been held as a sacred act. It was submitted to various physical or technical constraints such as the presence of water or the ability to defend the occupants against attack, but the determining factors for the selection or rejection of a site were often of a more subtle nature.

TOWN PLANNING

Settings

Most towns were built after a careful study of the characteristics of the land. The immeasurable qualities of the landscape, the mysterious patterns that lie within the countryside were analysed and defined. The perception and reinforcement of major features and important aspects have given birth to geometry (literally, measuring of the earth)[11] of the land whose lines relate different elements to one another. It was understood that the existing topography already has an underlying order.

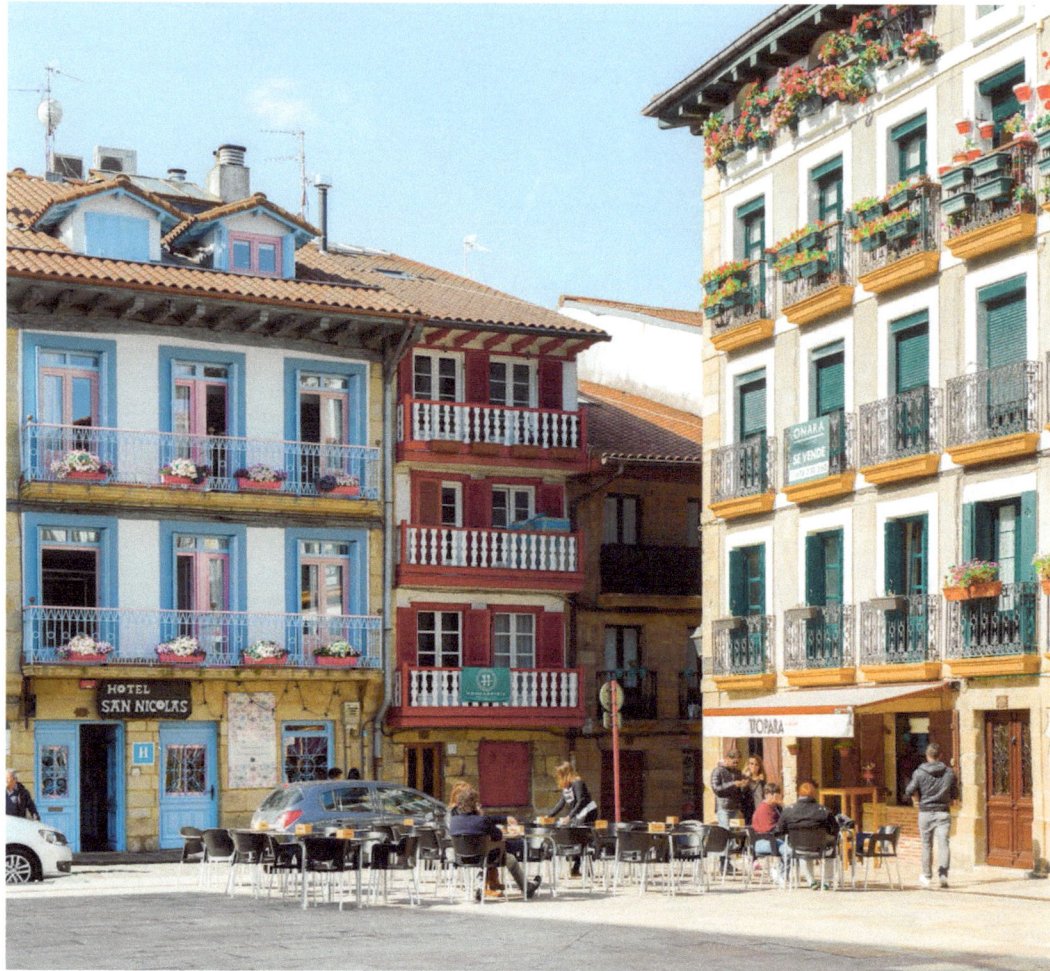

Town centres

The risk when defining a new town centre exclusively with technical constraints such as the distribution of services, power grid or traffic flow, is these considerations often dilute the symbolic significance of such a centre and disempower its function. In overlaying more than one important function onto the natural heart of the site as defined by its traditional or geographic significance, a feeling of belonging, of natural integration and a sense of purpose can be achieved. It will be as if the land itself was giving birth to the concept rather than having the concept arbitrarily imposed from the outside.

Various elements can be assembled in the town centre to strengthen it. Many settlements where originally built near a bridge, a point of convergence where local and transiting traffic flow can be channelled to increase the trade of the local business, it was also a very strong link, increasing the cohesion of a development.

A town square can be used for a variety of purposes at various times, as a market place for example, and a bus stop for public transport adds to the functional role of the centre. It should also have a recreational role, which can be achieved by coffee shops restaurants ... etc. and be close to park land.

For the town centre to be the hub of all activities it should be the junction of cycling and pedestrian paths traversing the site.

Finally, the town centre should fulfil a residential role, to avoid the "dead town centre syndrome" some residential areas should be planned in and around the centre.

Site focus

Traditionally the foundation of a city was closely related to the recognition and empowerment of the site focus, either with the erection of a sacred building or the planting of a tree for example. It was called the omphalos by the ancient Greeks, meaning - navel-, a pivot around which everything else revolves. The Romans called it the axis mundi, the axis of the world, connecting the energies of earth and heavens.

Its definition is akin to the stabilisation of the untamed energies of the Earth, it was the first step of civilisation on virgin land.

Nowadays the site focus can accommodate a tree, a park, a grove or some communal-use structure such as a public building.

51

12 Frances A.Yates -
The Art of Memory-
(The University of
Chicago Press 1966)

12 Giulio Camillo and
his adaptation of the
Vitruvian Theatre for
mnemonic purpose is at
the centre of the revival
of Vitruvius by Venetian
architects, especially
Palladio. The classical
theatre is reflecting the
proportions of the world.
The seven accesses to
the auditorium and the
five stage entrances
are determined by the
points of four equilateral
triangles inscribed within
a circle which centre
is the centre of the
orchestra. According
to Vitruvius, these
triangles correspond
to the trigons inscribed
by astrologers in the
circle of the zodiac. The
circular theatre is the
zodiac and the twelve
entrances are the twelve
signs connected by the
four triangles.

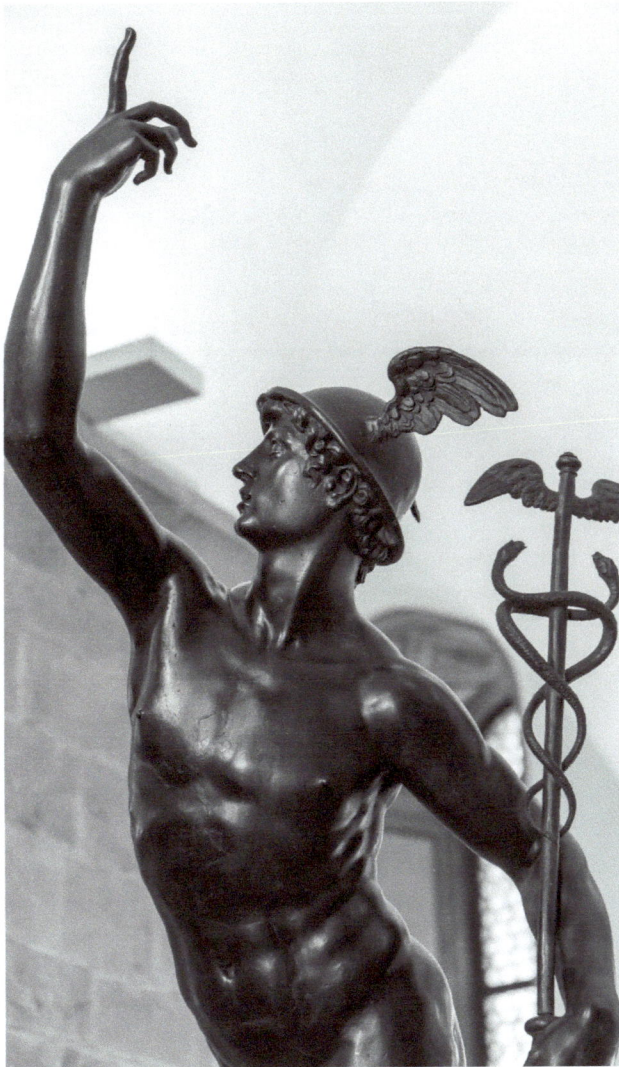

"I have read,
I believe in
Mercurius
Trismegistus, that
in Egypt there were
such excellent
makers of statues
that when they
had brought some
statue to the
perfect proportions
it was found to be
animated with an
angelic spirit. For
such perfection
could not be
without a soul..."

RESONANCE WITH THE UNIVERSE

THE SOUL OF THE HOUSE

Dame Frances A. Yates writes [12] "that in the Hermetic book The Asclepius, which was the theoretical basis for talismanic magic, the magical religion of the Egyptians is explained. They knew how to infuse the statues of their gods with cosmic and magical powers; through prayers, incantations and other processes they gave life to these statues, in other words they knew how to make gods. But more than prayers and incantations, the main factor which enabled these cosmic forces to reside in statues and buildings, or for them to acquire a "soul", was through the harmony of proportions.

This fact is confirmed by the discourse of Giulio Camillo [13] (1480-1544) about his Memory Theatre (A wooden theatre crowded with images and writings designed to assist and structure the memory of all things one could wish to store and remember) If a soul can be embodied in a statue, could it also be embodied in a house? The answer to this question is within us, it is part of our memory and part of our experience. It is a tenuous and delicate feeling that we all had when we were children, the sense of wonder exuding out of certain places.

I remember some houses, built with the same material as the rest of the town, designed in the same style to face the same climate and provide the same service as the houses surrounding them. The only difference being this indescribable sense of connection to the site and to people, generating a recognition, like a meeting with an old friend. They were designed and built with love and care by people who had a sense of proportion and a feeling for the site.

As we grow older, the places and building which awaken in us this sweet feeling of resonating with something higher and more beautiful than our daily life need to be more powerful.

MEASURES AND PROPORTIONS

Measures:

Since time immemorial units of measure have related to the human body, inches, feet and cubit, the distance between the elbow and the tip of the fingers.

It was in 1840 that the metric system was decreed as the official standard in France. The metre was defined as one ten-millionth of the distance between the equator and the North Pole. French scientists measured part of this distance, treating the Earth as a perfect sphere, and then they estimated the total distance which was in turn divided by ten million. After it was discovered that the Earth is not a perfect sphere a standard metre made of a bar of platinum iridium alloy was kept in Sevres near Paris.

In the 1960s the metre was defined as being 1650763,73 wavelengths of red light from a krypton 86 source.

Since 1983, the metre is the distance travelled by light in a vacuum in 1/299792458 of a second.

As we can see the metric system is a very artificial standard moving further and further away from a human reference. It does not consider, in its rigidity, the ever-changing nature of the universe in its diversity of expressions. The early standards varied from place to place, they were related to parts of the human body, inches and feet. Cubits were being used mainly for important and sacred buildings.

The word cubit is derived from the Latin -Cubitum- designating the ulna, the bone extending from the elbow to the wrist, opposite the thumb. It indicates a physical human measure.

Often this unit was much longer than the forearm of a normally constituted human being, and it is suggested that the calculation of its length was just the ratio of the human forearm with another measure of a different nature.

The cubit varied between 430mm and 560mm (17 to 22 inches). Even within a given culture in a specific area, different cubits could be used -the common cubit, the royal cubit slightly longer and the sacred cubit even longer.

The Greek, Etruscan and Roman cubit had a length of 444mm. The Celtic cubit used in Gaul was 523mm.

The Cambodian cubit or -hat- is 435mm and was the unit used to build Angkor Wat, the temple of Vishnu.

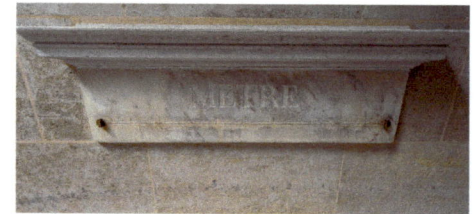

Standard meter

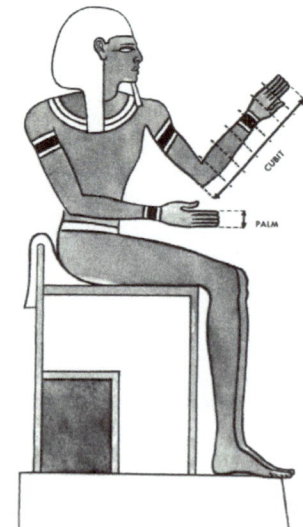

53

Plan for a house built in Albany, based on the "Vesica Pisces" using a cubit calculated from the latitude of the site. All the interlocked circles have a radius of 11 cubits. The fireplace is situated in the centre of the main circle.

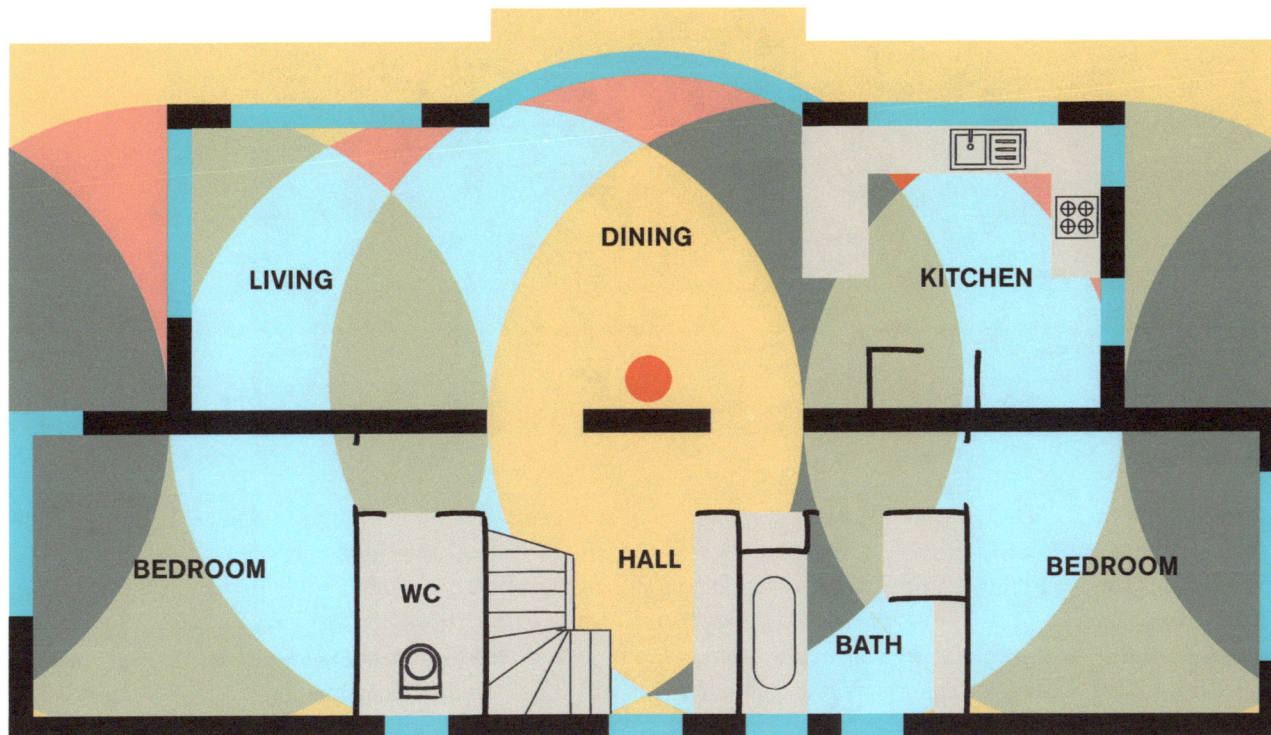

14 N. Pennick (The Ancient Science of Geomancy) CRCS Publications

15 N. Pennick (The Ancient Science of Geomancy) CRCS Publications

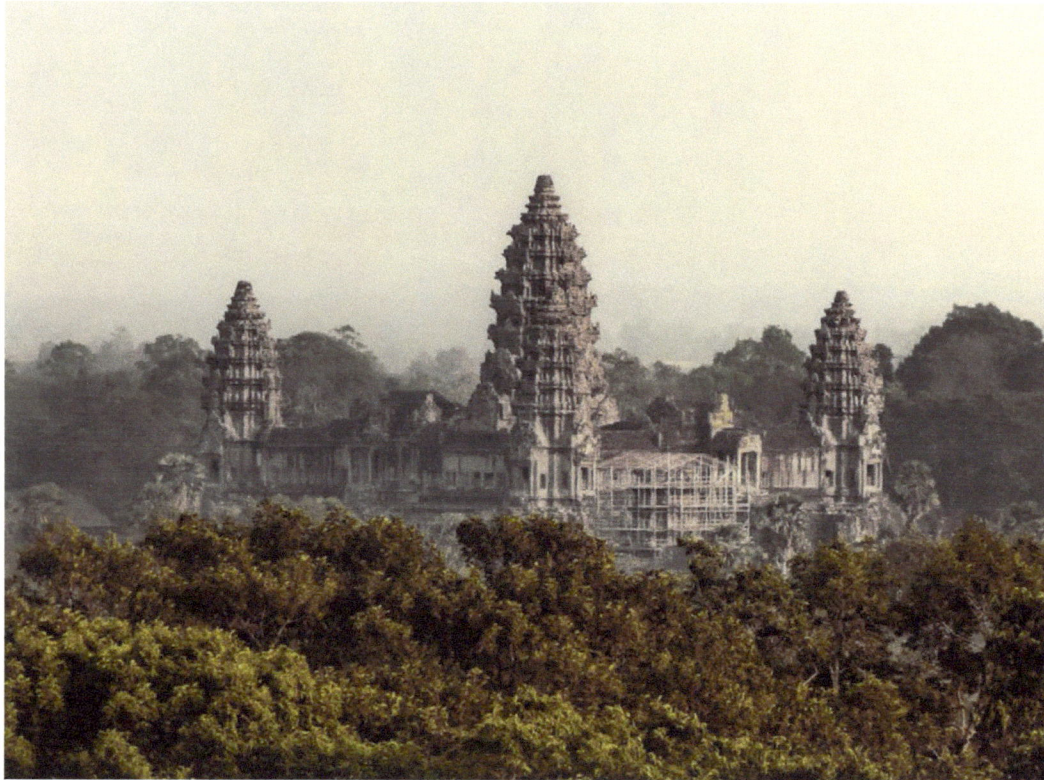

Angkor Wat

"All important parts of the temple are related to cosmological interval. In Hindu sacred history, there are four, time periods, or Yugas which together compose one cycle. They begin with a golden age, the Krita Yuga, and progress through Treta Yuga, Dvapara Yuga to the Kali Yuga. The last two periods are the worst, and the geomancers at Angkor have appropriately placed them at the furthest distance from the sanctuary. Thus, the vast rectangular moat which surrounds the whole temple has a width of 439 hat, symbolising the 432,000-year cycle of the Kali Yuga, the last and most decadent age of man. Incidentally, discrepancies between the temple's dimensions and the era lengths can be accounted for by the need to achieve the best fit between symbolic lengths and the astronomical alignment, which are of course fixed. From the first step of the western entrance gateway to the balustrade wall at the end of the causeway is 867 hat, symbolising the 864,000-year period of the Dvapara Yuga. Thence to the central tower is 1296 hat, corresponding to the 1,296,000 years of the Treta Yuga; and the distance between the first step of the bridge to the geomantic centre of the temple is 1734 hat, which represent the 1,728,000 year-period of the Krita Yuga."[14]

King's College Chapel in Cambridge, built by King Henry VI of England is one of the last Gothic churches to be erected by masons according to the old principles, embodying in its geometry the mysteries of the faith.

"Numerologically, the number 26 is dominant. There are 26 great stained-glass windows, 26 structural uprights, 26 ribs in each pair of fans in the stone vaulting, 26 apertures in each panel of side-chantry tracery, etc. The number 26 is a key symbol in cabbalistic gematria, a widely used symbolic system in which the letters in Hebrew or Greek were given number equivalents. In this way, a name can be symbolised by a length in any predetermined unit. Twenty-six represent the ineffable name of god, in Hebrew, JHVH."[15]

55

"The length of King's college Chapel is 288 feet, or 192 cubits. 192 is the gematrial number of the Greek MAPIAM, the name of the Virgin Mary, who is the principal patron of the college and its chapel.

The length is also equal to the sum of the two cabbalistic sephiroth, Hesed (72) and Gevurah (216), which represent respectively Mercy and Power."[16]

16 N. Pennick (The Ancient Science of Geomancy) CRCS Publications

17 J.-P. Dillenseger (Habitation et Sante) Dangles

In the cathedral of Strasbourg in Alsace, the unit of measure used is a length of 630mm which represent half the Polar axis of the Earth (12'712'178,377m) divided by ten million. 630mm being also the ideal dimension to design stairs (2 risers and 1 tread should add to 630mm). [17]

A building designed with a cubit in harmony with the site will act as a transformer and a resonator of cosmotellurian forces. The tellurian vibrations captured by the shapes and volumes are transformed for the benefit of man. When a building acts as a resonator it vibrates at the same frequencies as the environment and enhances them. Everyone must have experienced the phenomenon of resonance while singing or humming in a small space such as a shower or a bathroom, certain notes seem to set the whole space in vibration. Certain building's ability to resonate reaches far beyond the sound spectrum; they act as resonator for cosmotellurian forces as well.

We need thus to work out a cubit in relation to the latitude of the site rather than the metric system which is calculated according to the Earth's meridian. The latitude determines the site's exposure to solar and cosmic radiation.

The rotational speed of the earth on the equator is 40,000km/24 = 1666kph.

To know the speed on another parallel we need the cosine of the degree of latitude. If we take as an example the parallel situated 40 degrees north (or south) we can look up the trigonometric ratios for 40 degrees and find the value of the cosine which is 0.766. The speed of the earth at this latitude will be 0.766x1666= 1276kph.

We can then find out the perimeter of the earth at this latitude which is 1276x24= 30,624km.

If we use the same ratio used to define the length of a metre (1/10,000,000 of the quarter of the Earth's meridian) to define the length of a local cubit we will obtain: -30,624/4= 7656km or 7,656,000m which is then divided by 10,000,000 to obtain the value of 0.7656 (very close to 0.766, the cosine of 40 degrees). This indicates that one can also use the cosine of the site's degree of latitude to determine the length of a cubit in resonance with its geographic position.

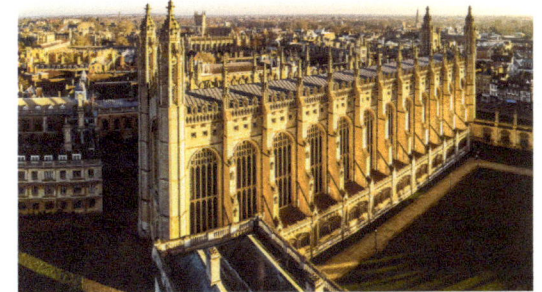

King's College

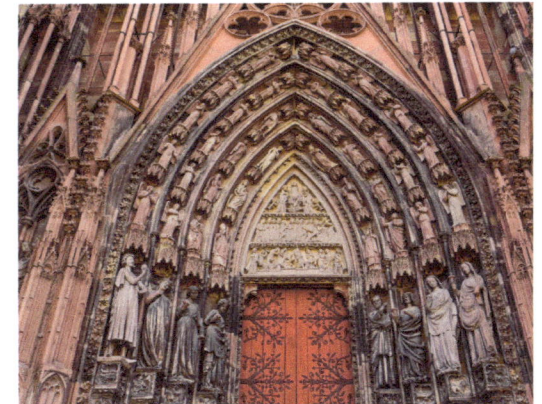

Strasbourg Cathedral

56

Proportions

Everything in nature indicates an underlying order, a regular pattern and harmony.

In the mineral world, the process of crystallisation, in its infinite diversity, always follows certain patterns according to each element.

The shape of leaves and their position on the stems follow a predetermined order particular to each species.

The growth of seashells and the horns of rams for example develop according to invariable mathematical blueprints.

In plants we often see leaves, seeds and fruit grow according to certain recurring patterns such as 1,2,3,5,8,13, etc. or 4,7,11,18,29, etc. called Fibonacci sequence, according to the work of Leonardo Fibonacci the Italian mathematician of the 12th century.

We often see leaves, seeds and fruits grow according to certain patterns.

In the Fibonacci series, each number in a sequence is the sum of the preceding two numbers. It is also interesting to note that the ratio between two numbers following each other in a Fibonacci series is approximately equal to the -golden mean- (1.618) and comes closer to it as the numbers grow.

The Fibonacci sequence is found everywhere in nature, from the arrangement of pads on cats' feet to organically produced spiral structures. The growth of certain plants follows a predetermined spiral pattern, where clockwise and anticlockwise spirals alternate with each other.

The artichoke leaves grow following five spirals in one direction and eight in the other. Its arrangement of leaves on the stem, or phyllotaxis, is 5/8, two numbers following each other in a Fibonacci series. The phyllotaxis of daisies is 21/34 and for the sunflower it is 55/89.

If a curve is drawn on which all the spirals of this series can be read. We can see that the angle formed by two successive points is constant and its value is 137 degrees 28 minutes. This value is also the result of 360 degrees divided by 1,618 (golden mean). It seems that the Golden section is more than just a tool to measure graphic and volumetric proportions; it is a constant in life's processes itself.

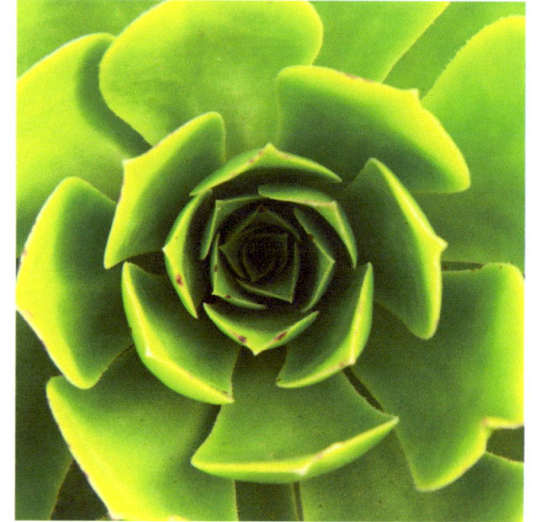

Phyllotaxis

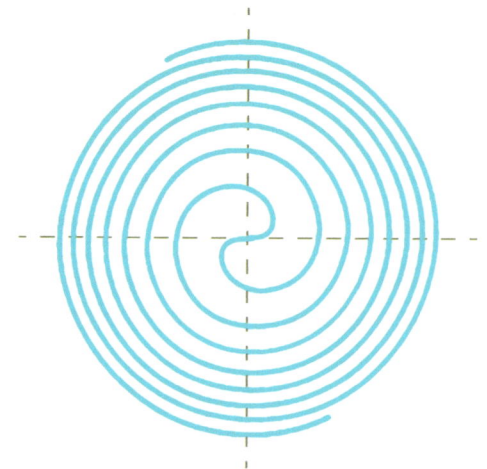

Double spirale

The arrangement of leaves on a stem follows a pattern generated by the Fibonacci number series.

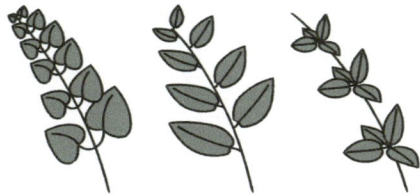

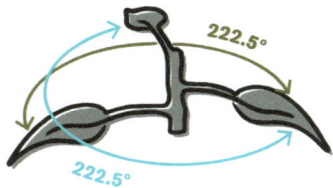

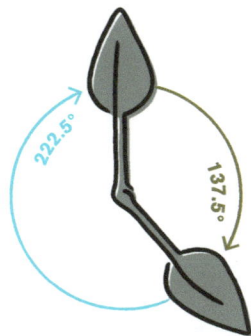

Plan and sacred geometry study for a rammed earth house in Dongara (Western Australia)

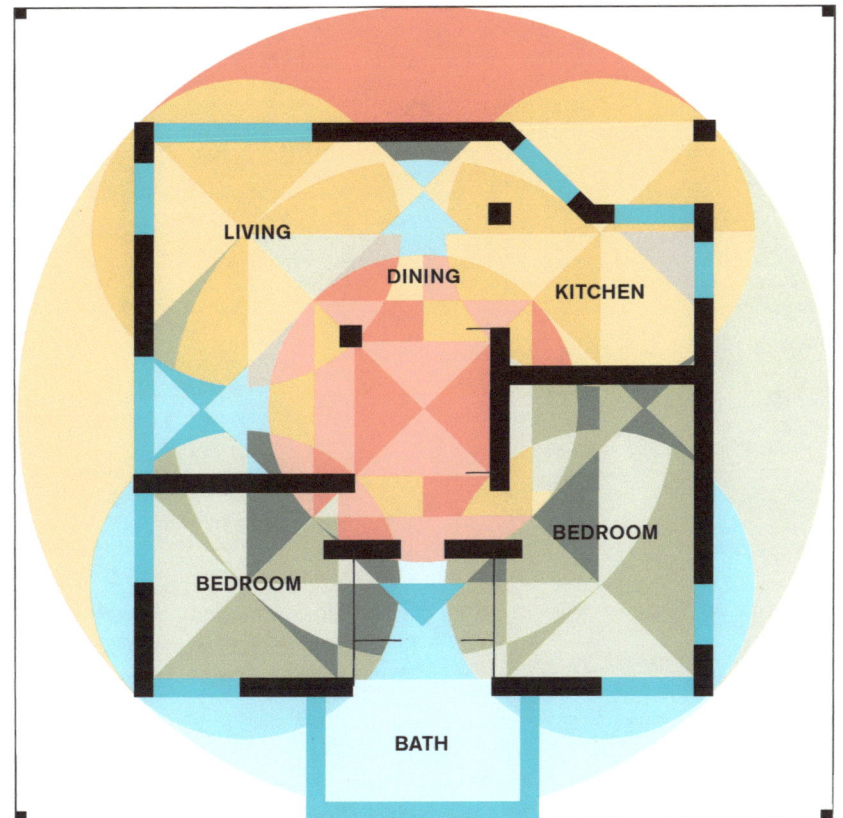

222.5°

222.5°

222.5°

137.5°

LIVING

DINING

KITCHEN

BEDROOM

BEDROOM

BATH

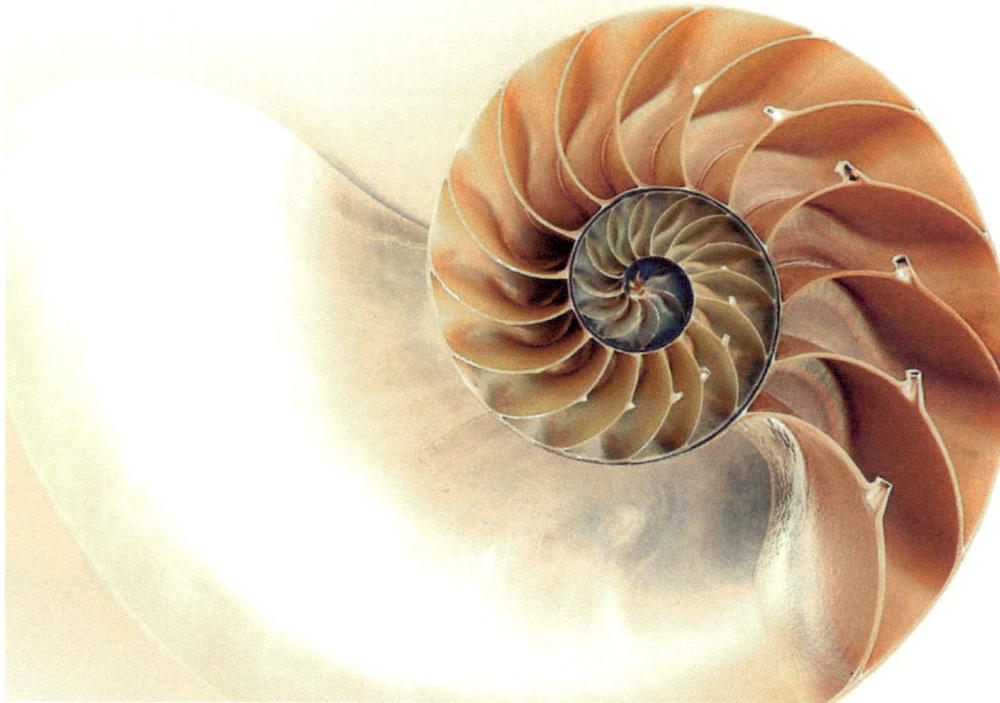

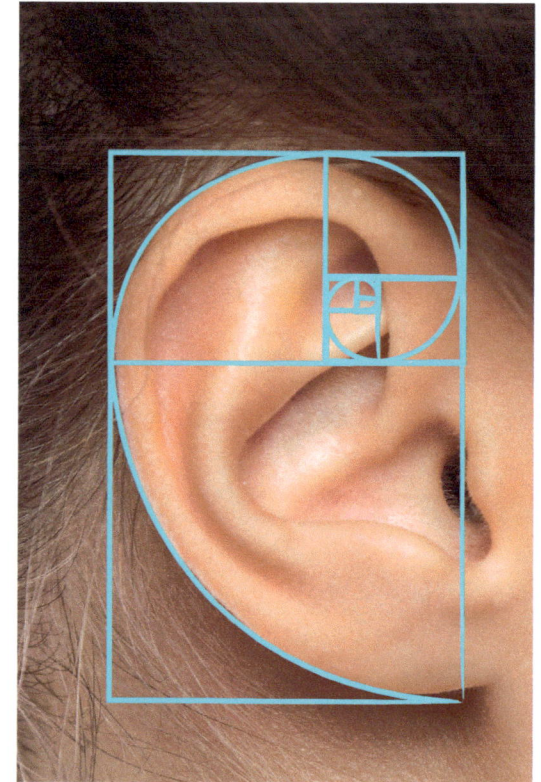

The Golden Mean spiral in which the geometrical increase of the radial arms is equal to 0.618 is found in the Nautilus Pompilius, the conch shell held in the hands of the Indian Divinity Shiva as a symbol of creation.

In the Golden Mean, also called Divine Proportion, a line is divided so that the ratio of the length of the small segment to the big segment is identical to the ratio of the length of the big segment to the total length of the line, this ratio or phi (f) has a mathematical value of 1.618.

This proportion is often encountered in nature. It is the blueprint for the growth of certain seashells, plants, animal and human embryos. It has been frequently used in architecture since antiquity, especially in Greek temples.

From the shape of galaxies to the shape of the human ear, we can observe forms in nature generated by the Golden Mean Spiral.

Measurements based on the human body:

Measurements were based on the human body, and were expressed in inches, feet and cubits. Architecture was then in resonance with the inhabitants.

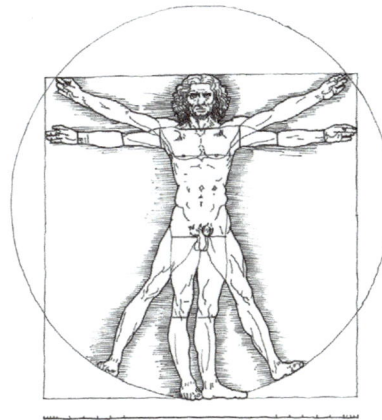

Leonardo da Vinci

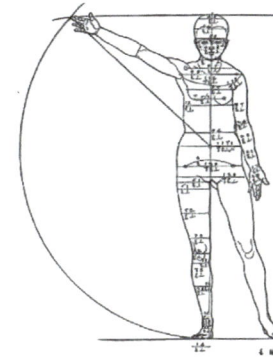

Vitruvius man

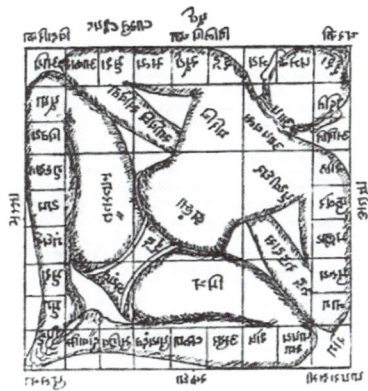

Vastu mandala used to trace the plan of cities and temples in India

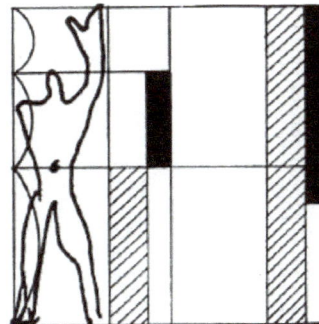

'The Modulor' Le Corbusier

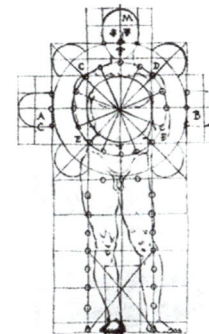

Di Gorgio

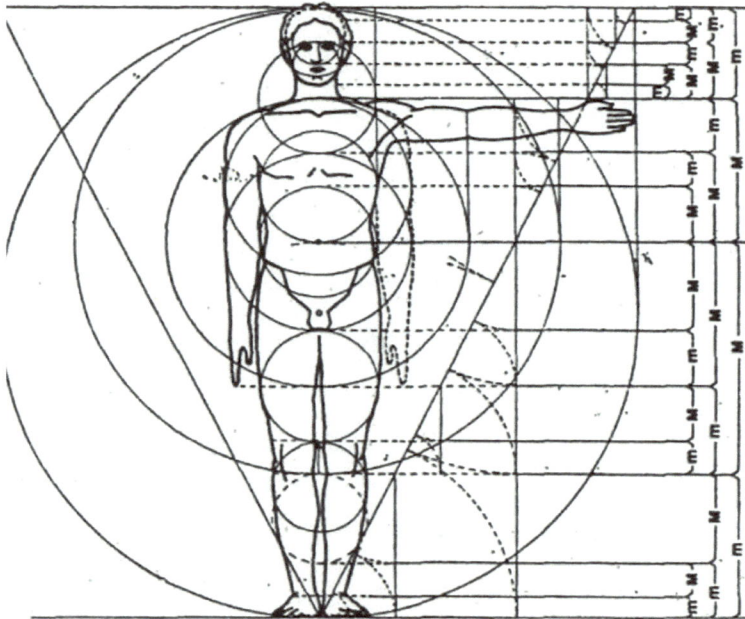

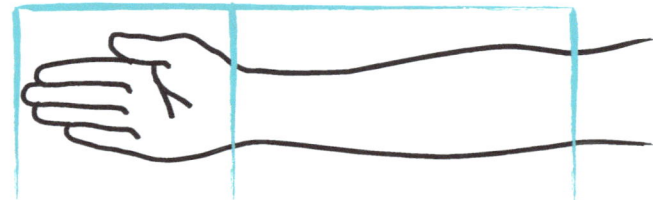

1 : **1.618** (approx)

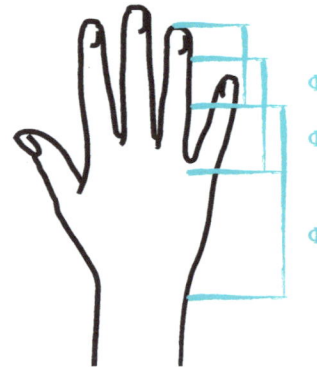

The human body is the primary standard of measure with which we measure the universe surrounding us, it is the reference and contains the blueprints of all manifested forms, it is like a tuning fork resonating with the whole universe

61

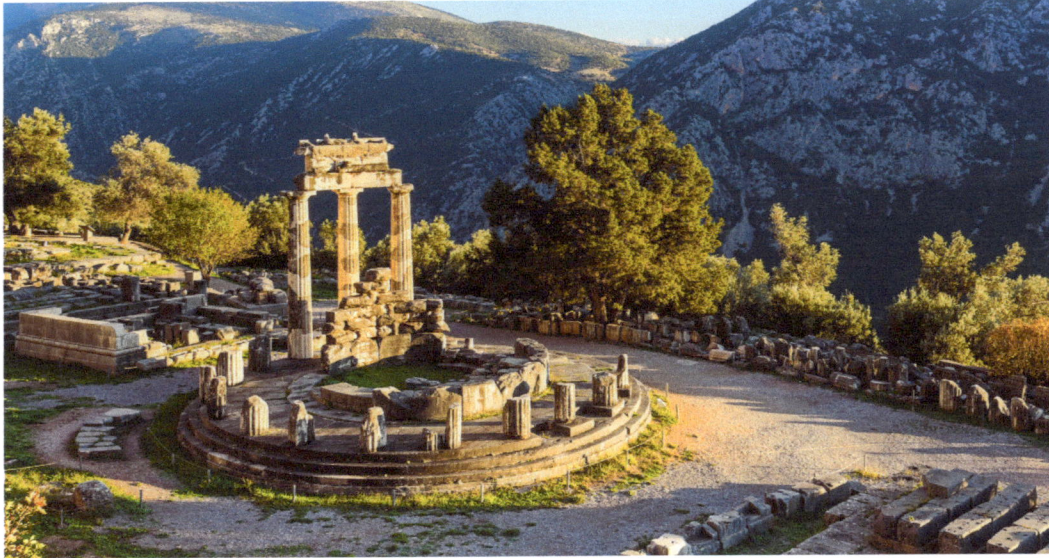

Sacred Geometry

Geometry is the study of the order of space, the measure of the relationship between space and forms. It is the knowledge of the laws governing the manifestation of abstract cosmic energies on Earth.

The circle: The circle is the most harmonious geometrical figure; each point of the perimeter is equal distance to the centre. It has symbolised perfection, God and the sun since the most ancient times. Of all plane figures having the same perimeter, the circle encloses the greatest area.

It has been used since the earliest times as a plan for tents, tepees, huts and houses, with the fire usually placed at the centre.

Sacred monuments and temples are often planed as circles, like Stonehenge and Greek and Roman temples.

The dome usually represented the world of spirit and the square the world of matter.

The square: The square is a stable and symmetrical figure and it symbolises the material world. Unlike the circle but like other regular polygons its orientation is important, usually according to the cardinal points. The angles act as form-fields transmitters and the sides as receptors.

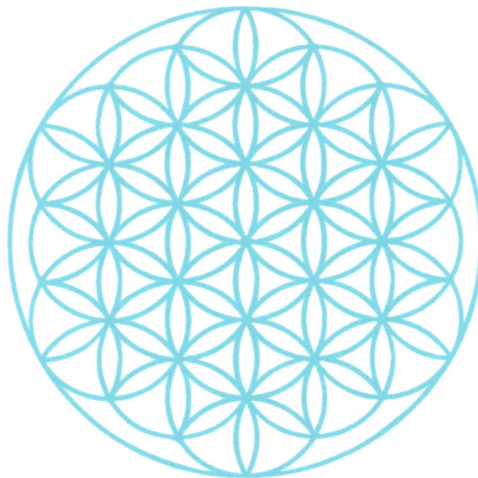

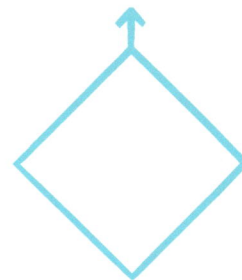

EMISSION

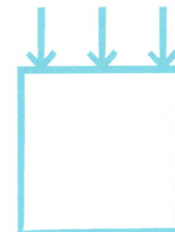

RECEPTION

62

The triangle: It is the symbol of the Christian Trinity (Father, Son, and Holy Spirit) as well as the Hindu Trinity (Brahma, Vishnu, Shiva). Of all the regular polygons, the angles of the triangle have the strongest form-field emission capacity.

An isosceles triangle whose base and height are the same size as the side of the square in which it is drawn - was used by the master cathedral builder to design the proportions of the Strasbourg Cathedral.

The isosceles triangle whose base is double the height has also been used to determine harmonious proportions.

The pentagon: The five-sided regular polygon generates the pentagram, a symbol of magic representing man when upright and the beast when inverted. The pentagram generates the golden section.

The hexagon: This regular polygon is the most efficient shape to cover an irregular surface. It is found in nature in beehives, while the eyes of insects are formed of light-sensitive organs grouped under a lens composed of an equal number of hexagonal prism shaped facets. Many elements crystallise in a hexagonal pattern.

The hexagon generates the Star of David which is known to neutralise the effects of other form fields.

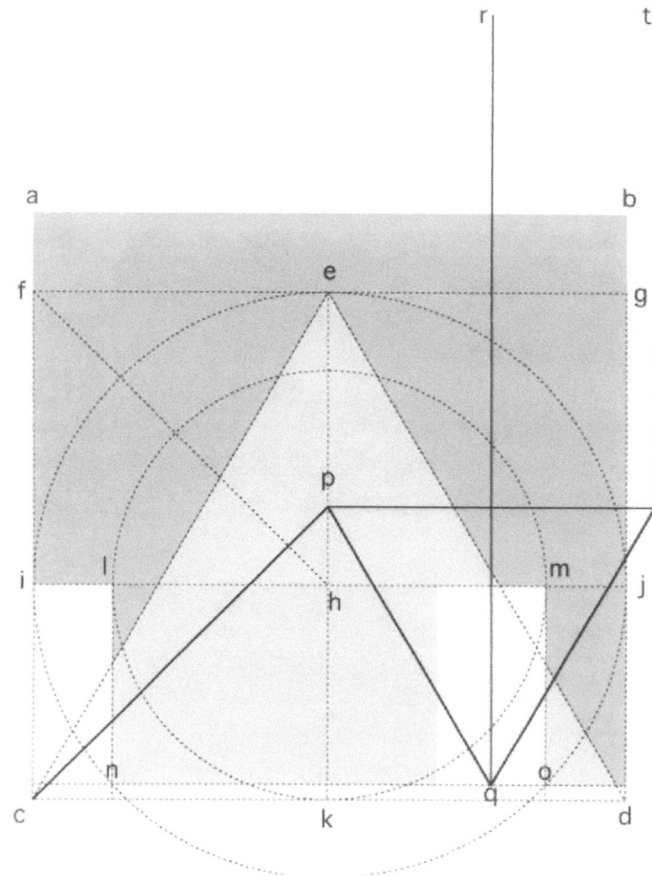

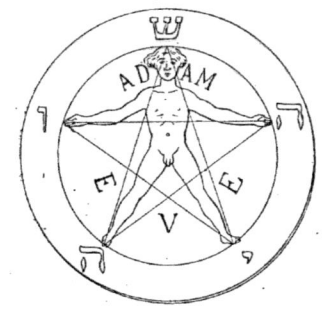

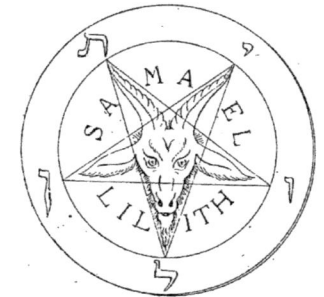

The octagon: In the cathedral of Speyer, in the south of Germany, the transition between the square plan and the dome is made by an octagon. This symbolic transition between heaven and earth was based on the octagon built with two squares oriented 45 degrees apart. This system was widely used in medieval architecture and is known as ad quadratum.

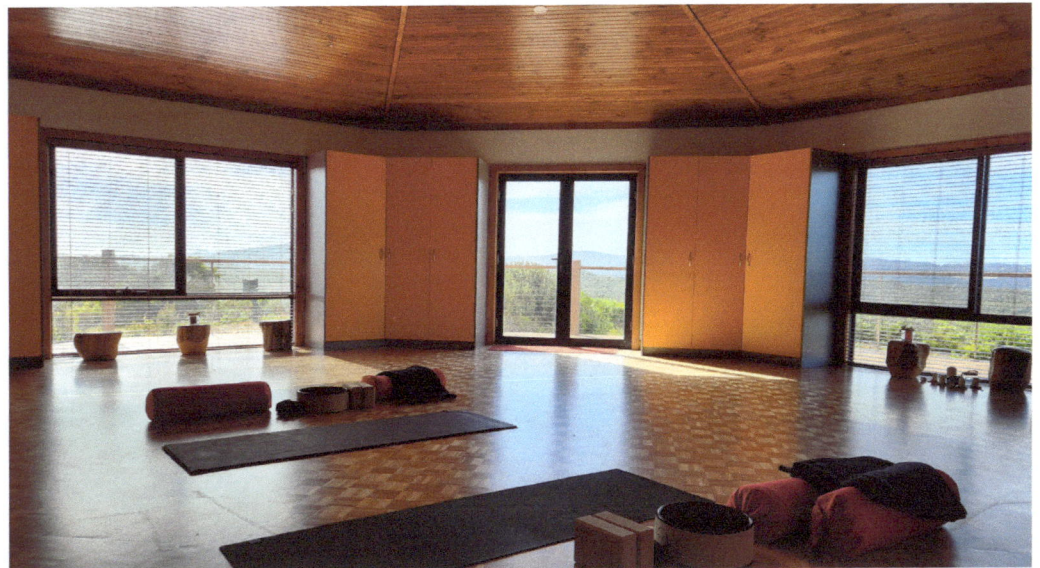

Octogonal yoga space, Denmark WA (Gobet-Hur Architects)

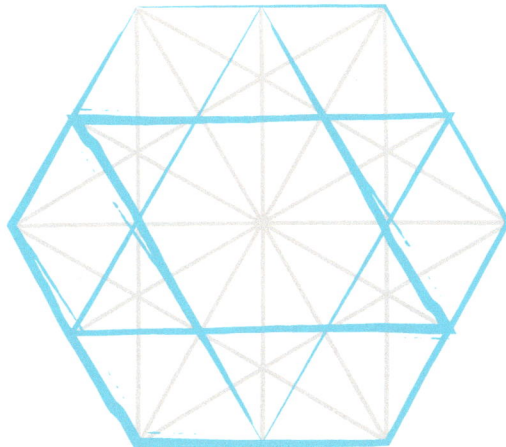

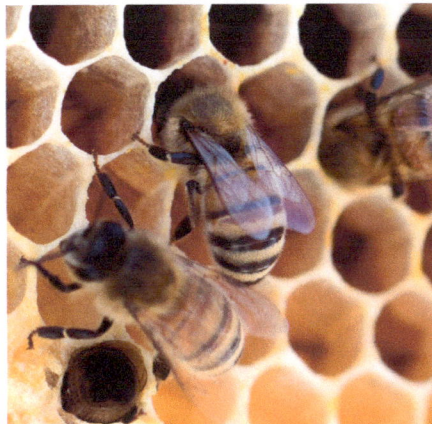

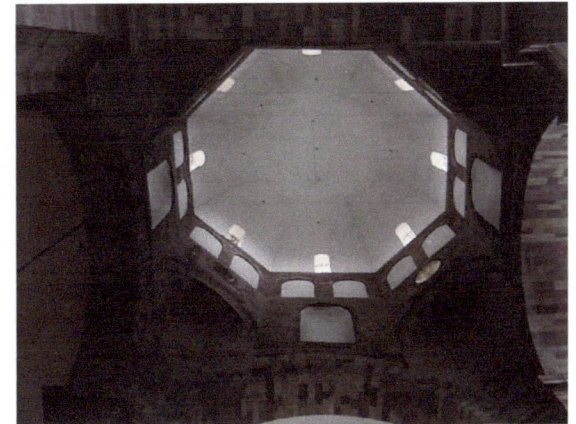

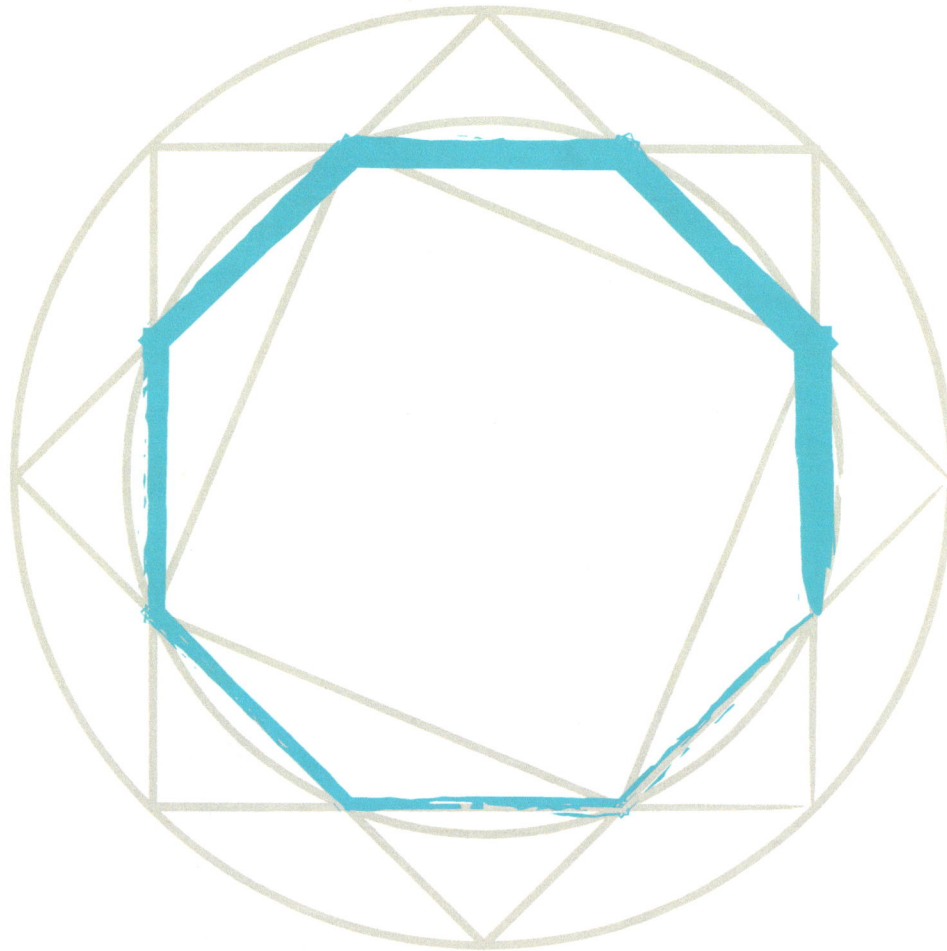

Ad quadratum, the process through which the material world transcends to the spiritual world through sacred geometry, from the square (material) to the circle or dome (spirit).

65

Sound and Geometry:

According to Pythagoras, all things are in essence mathematical numbers and can be represented by geometrical figures in different patterns.

The discovery of the relation between numbers and sound was very important. Vibrating strings generate musical intervals demonstrating a simple mathematical ratio relating to their length. When this ratio is 2/3, we obtain a fifth, and a major third when this ratio is 5/4.

For Pythagoras music reflected in the microcosm the laws which rule the cosmos as well as being a strong influence on our thoughts, emotions and actions.

The relation between sound and geometry is also shown in the experiment where sound frequencies cause random particles to assume various geometric patterns (Cymatics). This is how some violin makers test the shape and size of the wood to make a violin a resonating board.

These "musical" ratios were used extensively during the Gothic period; the cathedral builders were careful to design their buildings like finely tuned instruments of stone and glass in harmony with the music of the time.

"Music is liquid architecture; Architecture is frozen music"

– Johann Wolfgang von Goethe

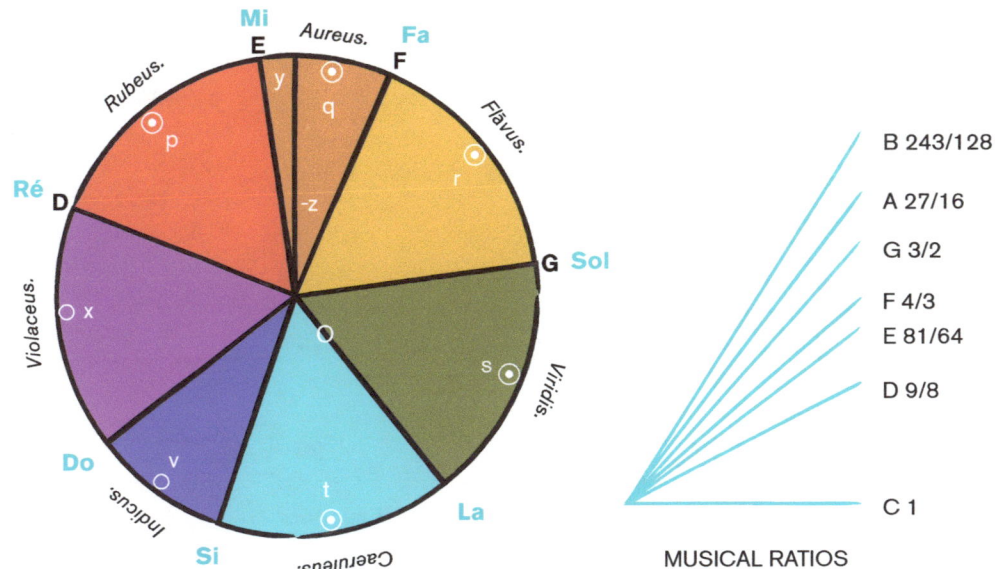

MUSICAL RATIOS

B 243/128
A 27/16
G 3/2
F 4/3
E 81/64
D 9/8
C 1

Chromatic Circle of Newton appeared in his work Opticks (1704). The colours (whose names are given in Latin) have been added.

66

18 Anil Ananthaswamy (Ancient sound waves sculpted galaxy formation) The New Scientist 30th March 2012

19 Dr. Hans Jenny (Cymatics- A Study of Wave Phenomena & Vibration) Macromedia Press 2001

20 Dr. Hans Jenny (Cymatics- A Study of Wave Phenomena & Vibration) Macromedia Press 2001

Cymatics:

From the first words of St. John's Gospel to the creating power of the "AUM" sound in the Vedic tradition, many creation myths in the world associate the act of creation with sound, such as the Australian creation myths relating how nature, plants and animals as well as humans, were sung into being.

In an article in "The New Scientist", Anil Ananthaswamy describes how: *"Sound waves that rang out in the early universe sculpted its structure. The best measurement yet of their imprint on galaxies is a boon to dark-energy studies."*[18]

The science of Cymatics, from the Greek ta kymatika, "matters pertaining to waves", shows the direct relation between geometric shapes and sound.

The name was coined by Hans Jenny, a Swiss doctor born in 1904 in Basel and a disciple of Rudolf Steiner. He taught for four years at the Rudolf Steiner School in Zurich. He spent most of his life practicing medicine in Dornach, a village near Basel where Rudolf Steiner built the Goetheanum, the world centre for the Anthroposophical Society.

Dr Jenny used a metal plate connected to an oscillator, a frequency generator will emit sounds to vibrate materials such as quartz sand, metal filings, fine powder or fluids to create patterns, these shapes change according to

the frequency and intensity of the sound. In Dr Jenny's film, "Cymatics- Bringing Matter to Life with Sound", we can see the appearance of geometric, floral and even animal like patterns, such as a snake like skeleton undulating in a viscous fluid.

Dr Jenny developed the Tonoscope in order to study the effect of the human voice on different materials and observe the difference between the human generated sounds and the mechanically generated sounds -organized patterns and configurations are quite apparent. They are there for the eye, man's most sensitive organ of sense, to see. A pattern appears to take shape before the eye and, as long as the sound is spoken, to behave like something alive. The breath alone can cause it to move; a texture of forms is created by the fluctuations of the voice. The eye can also see variations as the voice is raised or lowered. During continuous speech the patterns metamorphose continually."[19]

The patterns generated by the human voice are more alive and in constant flux, as the intensity of the breath varies. Furthermore, the same sounds will generate similar recognisable patterns with small variations associated withindividual voice characteristics.

The geometry of a well-designed space will resonate with the human body and act as a healing device.

As John Beaulieu (ND PhD) explains in his "Commentary on Cymatics":

"In energy medicine, the underlying vibrational field is called an energy field. The health practitioner seeks to perceive, evaluate, and support the energy field rather than focus on a specific symptom. The practitioner's goal is to use therapeutic modalities such as music, sound, touch, homeopathy, acupuncture, tuning forks, voice, and colour, to effect and change the energy field. As the person shifts into resonance with a more coherent field, their array of symptoms may disappear as a more harmonious pattern emerges. The idea of energy fields is both new and ancient. Physicists have sought to explain the strange behaviour of quantum particles through the existence of a unified field. "We may therefore regard matter as being constituted by the regions of Space in which the field is extremely intense...There is no place in this new kind of physics both for the field and matter, for the field is the only reality." (Albert Einstein)[20]

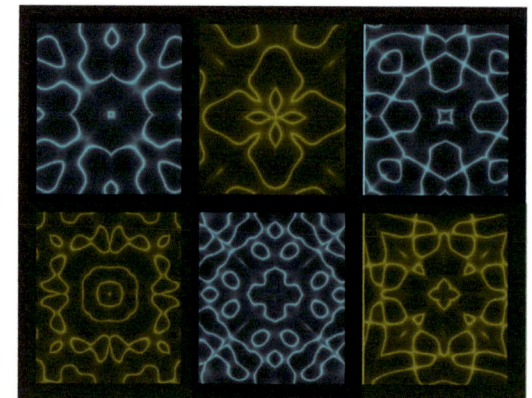

67

"In the beginning was
the Word and the Word
was with God and the
Word was God."

– John 1:1

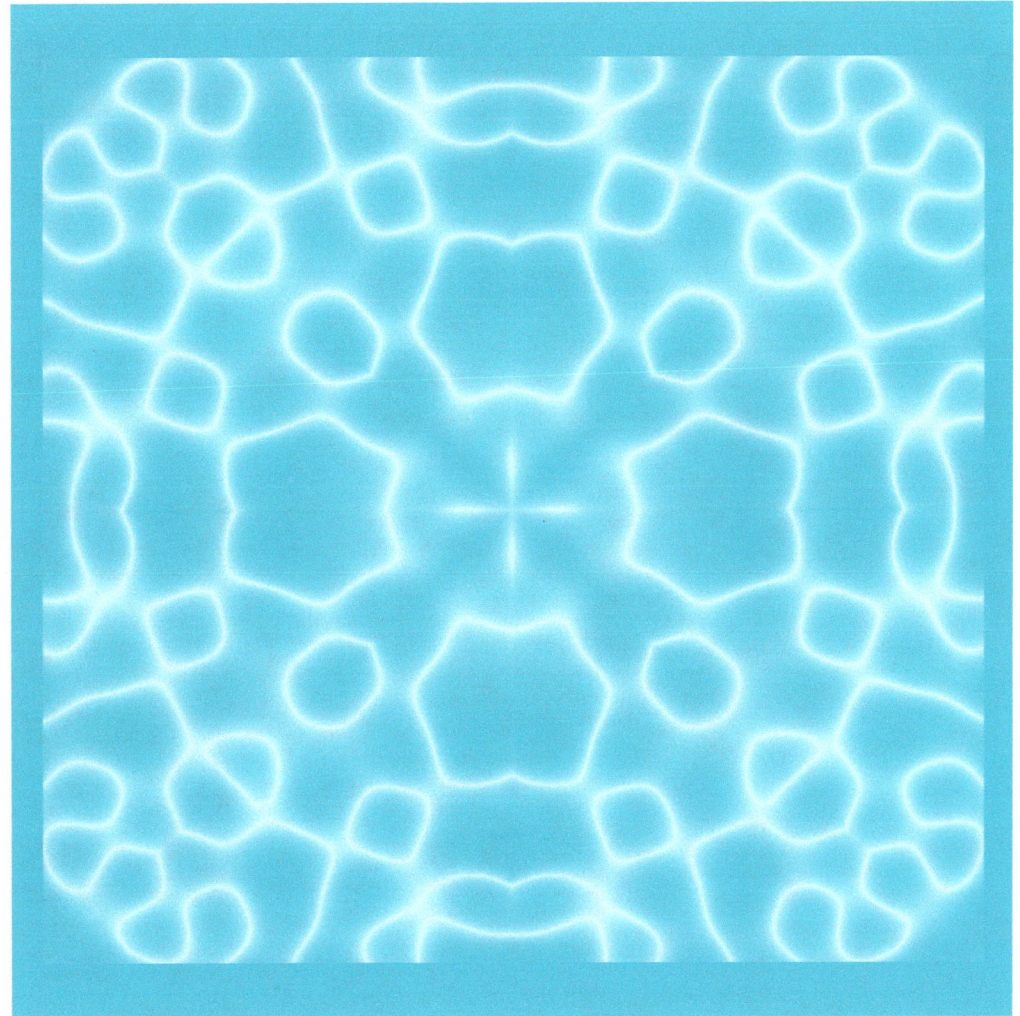

RESONANCE WITH THE CLIMATE

Architecture could be defined as a response to a local climate, through the availability of materials, experience and the acquisition of new skills to provide a durable and comfortable space.

Industrialisation and the availability of relatively cheap energy has enabled societies to diverge from these basic principles to provide cooling and heating mechanically instead of the traditional principles of passive solar design relying mostly on orientation, shading, ventilation and building mass.

During the last forty years, we have slowly come to realise that these principles are the necessary tools to turn back the effects of global warming and the increasing costs of energy.

High tech solutions are constantly being developed and while they are relevant in certain areas with high density construction or extreme climates, they are for the most part more expensive and often energy hungry throughout their life cycle.

It is now imperative to first gather all the data pertaining to a particular site, especially sunshine, prevailing winds and seasonal changes before proceeding with the design.

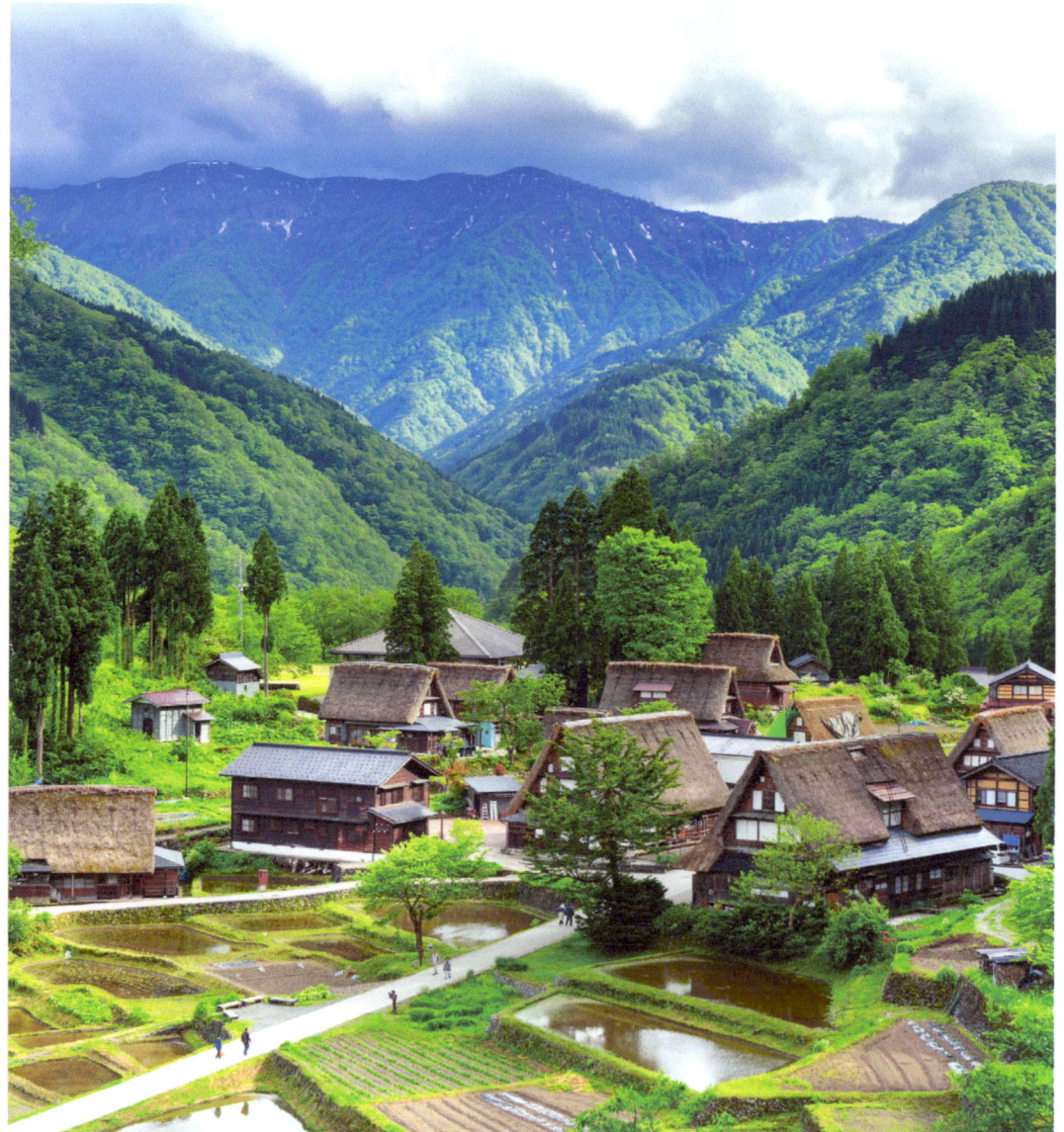

69

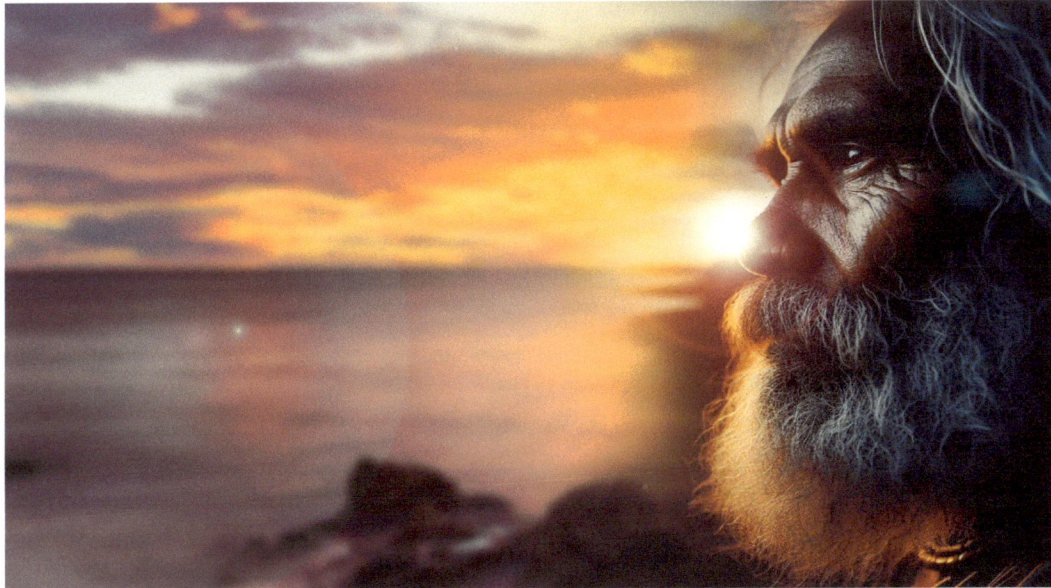

Wungud is the untouchable creator from which we all come. We come from water, this is where all Spirit comes from. Wungud infuses life through water, it reflects life into being.

RESONANCE WITH THE SITE

Positioning on the site

More often than not the position is restricted to a small area within the legal setbacks and street alignment. It is however possible even in an urban context to find and plot the geomagnetic grid, so the house can be designed according to the position of the knots and neutral zones.

The Local Tradition

Most people in industrialised societies have lost the deep connection to the land which characterised ancient cultures. By looking through the eyes of the last traditional cultures we may be able to remind ourselves of this connection. David Mowaljarlai is an Aboriginal elder from the Kimberleys, in the north west of Australia and he shares with us his people's vision of the land.

-Wungud is the untouchable creator from which we all come. We come from water, this is where all Spirit comes from. Wungud infuses life through water, it reflects life into being.

What is our relationship to the land according to Aboriginal culture? Before its birth the child tells his/her Mother who he/she is, its name, its nature, whether it is cloud, stone or plant ...etc.

For us ecology is relationship, kinship with the land. Nobody lives outside this Wunan, this law. Nothing can survive outside relationship, one is an unviable state in life. Western culture is a manifestation of the power of one, Aboriginal law is about relating, the relationship between Wodoi, hunted food or the male principle and Jungun, gathered food or the female principle. Men's business is outside, they observe, they create technologies. Women's business is inside, it is about gestation and nurturing. Men see what they see and Women see what they experience. We did not make these symbols, they were here in the land for all eternity.

70

21 (Transcript of a meeting with David Mowaljarlai in Bicton WA in January 1997)

22 Eilert Ekwall (The Concise Oxford Dictionary of English Place Names) Clarendon Press

23 James R. Tyrrell (Australian Aboriginal Place Names and their meaning) Simmons Ltd. Glebe Sydney 1933

This place, Moanna is a place where we get energy to increase our strength, it is an untouchable place. The land feeds you, the scenery feeds you and changes you. We are the reflection of the place we were conceived and/or born in. The place names the child and the child is born of the energy of the place. The relationship between the place and the child is inseparable. The land and us, are reflections of each other. The child becomes then the caretaker of the land of its birth and nobody can enter without its permission.-

To further explain the power of the land David Mowaljarlai tells the story of a woman, a lawyer from Sydney who came to the Kimberleys. *-She was infertile and was taken by Aboriginal women to a Wungud rock for a ceremony of fertility. As they were picking water lilies in a pond, the woman was bitten in the bum by a leach. That night she was woken up by a nightmare, she dreamt of a leach entering her womb. Now she is six months pregnant. The Wungud rock is vibrating and pulsating. We should look at Nature with receiving eyes.-*[21]

With common sense

It is easy to define the potential problems and disturbances on the grossest level, though, surprisingly, some people still fall in the same trap time and time again. The low price of a site will never make up for the damage it could cause to one's health. One should avoid sources of atmospheric, acoustic, electromagnetic, geologic and even visual pollution such as freeways and highways, high power lines and transformers, radar and microwave transmission towers and polluted industrial areas.

We should then look at the qualities the site has to offer, its topography, its orientation, its situation and the visual qualities of the surroundings. Whether it is a natural or a built environment does not matter as long as it is pleasing to the eye.

The best sites are oriented towards the south-west direction in the Northern Hemisphere and towards the north-west in the Southern Hemisphere.

It is advisable to have some knowledge of the geological nature of the area in general and of the site in particular. One can thus avoid geological faults and underground water currents.

The healthiest building site are on limestone, sand or chalk. Sites composed of clay, marl, peat, landfilled areas and creeks which have been filled should be avoided.

The name of a site can also give us a good indication of its history and quality. Names like **Morpeth** (Northumberland, UK) which literally means "murder path", **Maybole** (Strathclyde, UK) meaning "plain of danger", **Leith** (Lothian, UK) meaning "moist", **Skinburness** (Cumberland, UK) meaning "fortified place haunted by a demon" or **Malpas** (Cheshire, UK) meaning "bad pass" would suggest that the quality of the sites might not be best suited to build on.

Places such as **Greetland** (Yorkshire, UK) "gravelly land" or **Beauvale** (Nottinghamshire, UK) "beautiful vale" might be more suitable.[22]

Celtic names all over Europe would suggest an even better knowledge of the nature of the site. This knowledge would also be found virtually untainted in places like Australia where Aboriginal place names come from an intimate connection to the site. There, we find revealing names such as **Yweagre** "a miserable place" (NSW), **Yeo Yeo** "devil devil" (NSW), **Towalba** "a swamp" (WA), **Jindera** "haunted mountain" (NSW), **Micabit** "struck by lightning" (NSW), **Youlbung** "water scarce" (NSW) or **Windalup** "a permanent stream" (WA), **Taronga** "a beautiful view" (NSW), **Akoomie** "very good" (NSW) and **Quinbalup** "a happy place" (WA).[23]

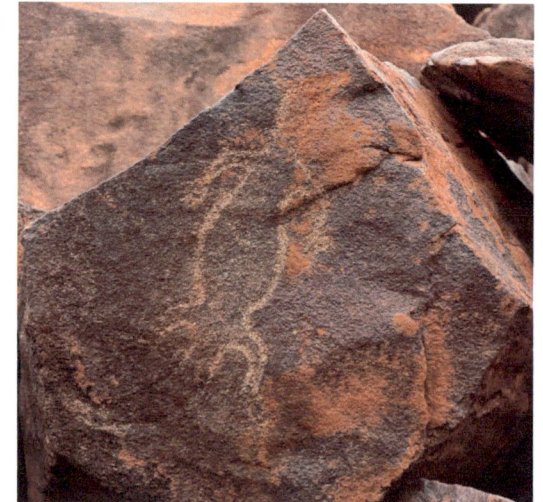

71

24 Souls on Fire,
Portraits and Legends
of Hasidic Masters (Elie
Wiesel)

I remember hearing the story of an old builder who was about to retire declaring how glad he was to stop working, since, according to him there was no more good land to build on. This was in the early 70s, in Switzerland, in an area where new houses are popping up every year! It illustrates the fact that suitable land to build on is becoming very scarce in big cities.

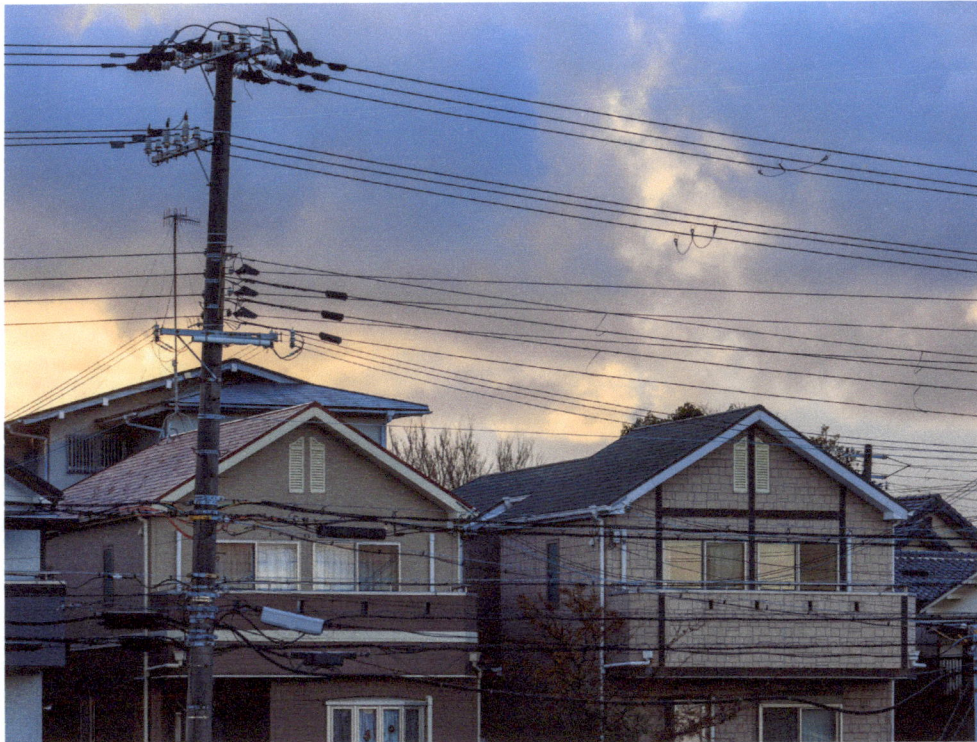

Events of great significance seem to create deep impressions on the fabric of the space-time continuum, they seem to impregnate a site with their energy which ripples in all directions.

Elie Wiesel (Nobel Prize for Peace) tells the story of a Hassidic rabbi travelling in the Polish countryside with his disciples at the end of the nineteenth century. [24]

The little group stopped late one night at a lonely train station. They were looking for accommodation and found beds in the local inn.

In the middle of the night the rabbi woke up in panic. He woke up all his disciples and told them to pack up. "We should leave immediately", he said, "This place is evil!". As they passed by the train station one of the disciples noticed the name of the village written on the wall, Oswizin, Polish for Auschwitz.

RESONANCE WITH THE LOCAL MATERIALS

Materials found or made locally are in harmony with the local conditions, and builders have the knowledge to work with them. They are ecologically and economically preferable to materials which must be transported long distances.

RESONANCE WITH THE LOCAL SKILLS

Architecture is more than the design of plans and elevations, the quality of the execution is as important, if not more. Traditionally workers on a building site were masters and companions, men who had studied the traditions, the skills and the secrets of their profession for many years. They had a kind of holographic perception of the art of construction, where each part had knowledge of the whole.

This was illustrated by the story of the bishop visiting the building site of a cathedral, long ago. When asking some worker what he was doing, the answer was not "I'm carving a stone "or "I'm mixing mortar", but "I'm building a cathedral". The architect himself came from the long learning process of apprenticeship through stone masonry and carpentry.

These professions where anchored in both heavens and earth. They had perfected their skills to the point of being real artists and their theoretical knowledge was supported by their esoteric wisdom.

Their chief motivation was the love of their art.

It is more difficult nowadays to find tradespeople with both excellent skills and a philosophy of life-giving importance to the wellbeing of others.

An appropriate design will consider the level of skills provided locally. It is unfortunately increasingly difficult to find tradespeople working with traditional methods and materials.

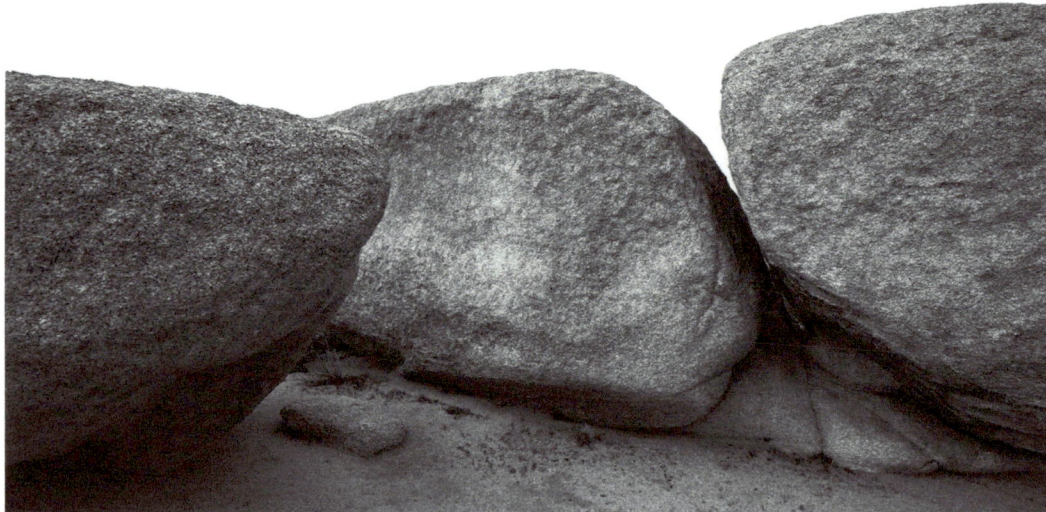

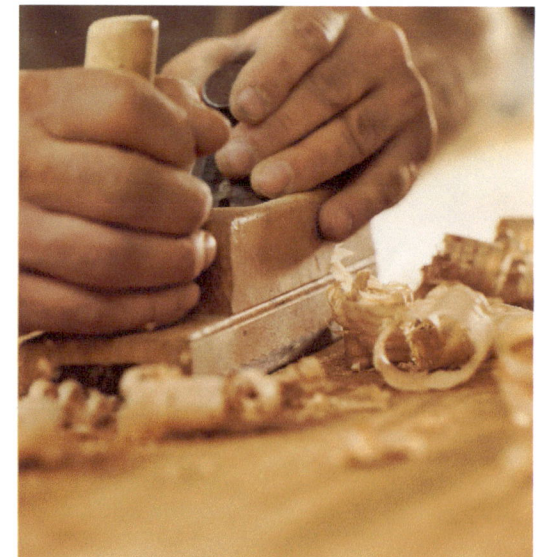

the art of building has been impoverished by industrialisation.

RESONANCE WITH THE INHABITANTS

The design of a house, the size of the rooms, the number of windows, the colours and the materials have a profound influence on our physical and psychological health. Within the same environmental context, different design solution will be expected for different types of people. The problem is to define what psychological category fits a given design solution. Our morphology, the shape of our body, is a good indicator of the type of house that will suit us best.

Morphopsychology gives us a better knowledge of ourselves; it defines four main psychological types of human beings. There is of course no pure type we are all a combination of the four, however we do have a dominant trait. The four types are defined as sanguine, choleric, phlegmatic and melancholic according to the ancient Greek tradition (Hippocrates).

Other system of type classification can be used to the same effect. Be it the "Four temperaments" according to Rudolf Steiner, the three "Doshas" according to the traditional Ayurvedic principles or the four humors and personalities defined by Hippocrates, shown on the table below.

The examples given above illustrate the importance of designing to satisfy needs that are sometimes not expressed but nevertheless inherent to the personality. What is sometimes considered as merely a matter of taste is often a deep need to feel protected in an environment suited to the way we view reality. In a couple, for example, one of the partners might choose or decorate a house exclusively according to his or her needs and taste. In such a situation, the other partner might feel alienated, literally without a home, without protection and without a place to be regenerated.

HUMOR	BODY SUBSTANCE	PRODUCED BY	ELEMENT	QUALITIES	COMPLEXION AND BODY TYPE	PERSONALITY (BROAD OUTLINE)
SANGUINE	BLOOD	LIVER	AIR	HOT AND MOIST	SANGUINE, MEDIUM FRAME, OVAL FACE	SOCIAL, OPTIMISTIC, CAN BE IRRESPONSIBLE
CHOLERIC	YELLOW BILE	SPLEEN	FIRE	HOT AND DRY	COMPACT-LEAN	ACTIVE, CAN BE SHORT TEMPERED
PHLEGMATIC	PHLEGM	LUNGS	WATER	COLD AND MOIST	CORPULENT	RELAXED, PEACEFUL CAN BE SLUGGISH
MELANCHOLIC	BLACK BILE	GALL BLADDER	EARTH	COLD AND DRY	MELANCHOLIC: SMALL FRAME	INTROSPECTIVE, SENTIMENTAL, GLUTTONOUS

74

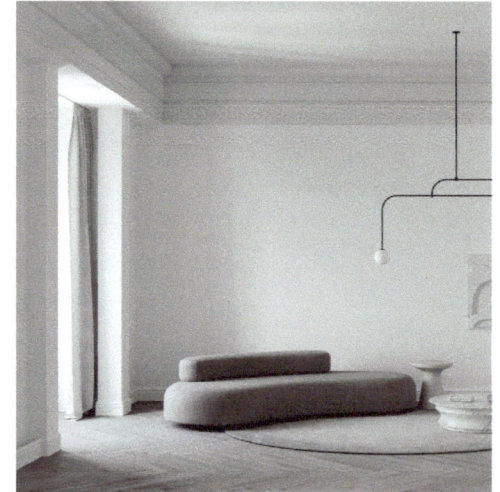

Sanguine Morphology

(Air)

The physical characteristic of this type are a triangular face, narrow chin, narrow chest and shoulders.

They like to dream; they are intellectual, idealistic and can be unstable and pessimistic. They need change.

Their house must be light and airy with great windows. They like Scandinavian furniture. Tidiness is not a priority.

Their preferred spaces are the study and the meditation room. Their colours are violet and white, the latter being predominant. For this type, chairs are not necessary a tatami or a meditation pillow will do.

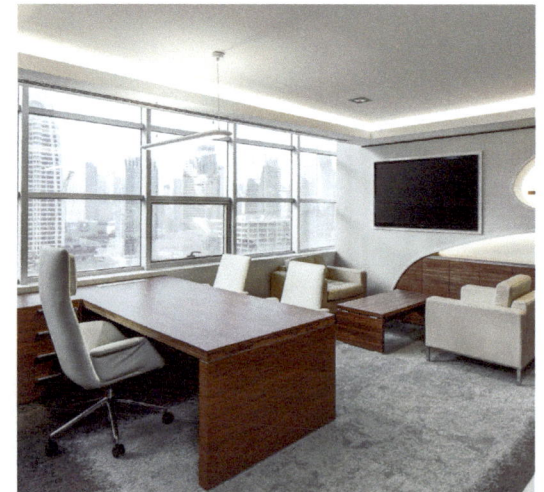

Choleric morphology

(Fire)

The physical characteristics of this type are a square face, olive skin, wide forehead, strong chin and jaw and wide shoulders. They like action and are active, impulsive and can be impatient. They need activity.

Their house must be functional and practical. Everything must be tidy and well organised. The decoration is subdued and without excess.

Their preferred spaces are the kitchen, the office and the work-shop. For them colours do not matter so much

For this type, chairs should be functional.

▽

Phlegmatic morphology

(Water)

The physical characteristics of this type are a round face, pink skin and a little round belly.

They like to communicate; they are clever and lighthearted and can be prone to excess. They need to exhibit.

Their house is like an exhibition, it gives them the opportunity to show off their furniture and light fittings. The decoration is often excessive.

Their preferred spaces are the living room and the dining room and their colours are orange and yellow.

For this type, chairs should be beautiful.

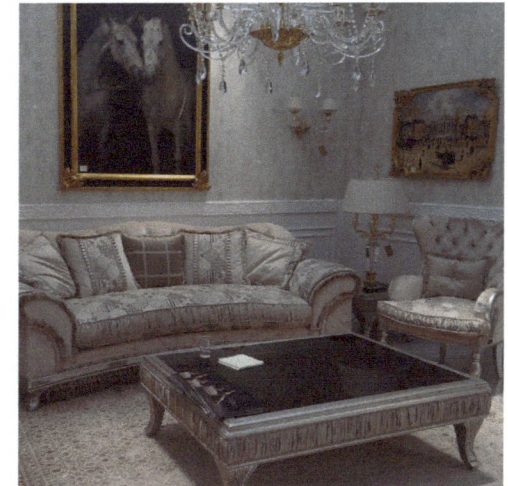

▽

Melancholic morphology

(Earth)

The physical characteristics of this type are wide lower face, double chin, big cheeks, pale skin and round belly.

They like to enjoy life; they are conservative, careful and can be timorous. They need security.

Their house must be solid and comfortable. They like antiques, tapestries and carpets, indirect lighting. Their preferred space is the living room -preferably near the fireplace and their colours are blue, brown and Bordeaux.

For this type, chairs should be comfortable.

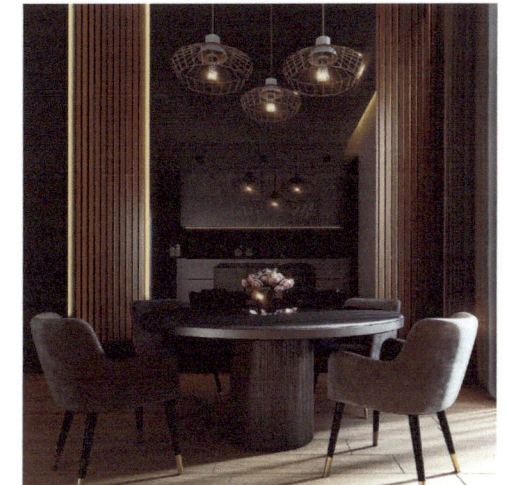

06 /
The Materials

77

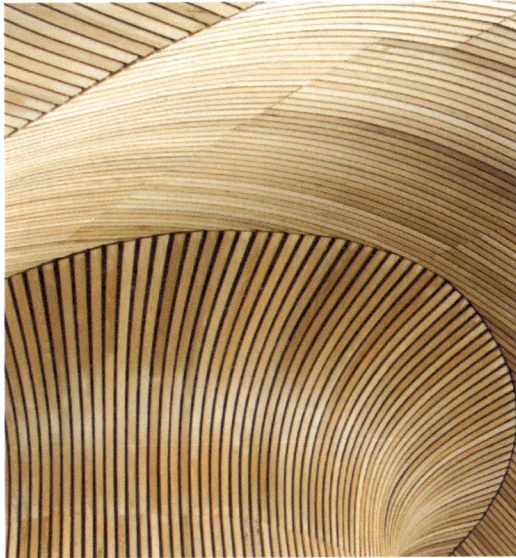

QUALITY

The quality of building materials is one of the most influential factors in a geobiological construction; the term "bioconstruction" can also be used. There are different criteria to define the suitability of materials.

Are they chosen for the benefit of the inhabitants and will they enhance the quality of their lives?

Every year new materials come on the market but, unlike pharmaceutical products, there is no rigorous testing to prove they are not toxic. In fact, you can buy some products clearly defined as poison, with the "Jolly Roger" symbol printed on the package, and use it anywhere in your house. This is usually the case for some paints, thinners, glues and insulating foams. How is this possible knowing that some people especially young children can spend up to 24 hours a day in their house and this environment is not safe!

With the development of modern transport, it is now possible to buy virtually any product from anywhere. A more ecological and sound way to build is to use local material.

It is now generally accepted that building materials have a determining influence on the health of the inhabitants as well as the environment.

The characteristics of materials suitable for a healthy house are the following:

- Permeability to gases to allow the building to breathe.

- No emission of toxic gases and radio activity.

- Good circulation of cosmotellurian energies.

- Good quality of acoustic and thermal insulation.

- Should not accumulate static electricity.

- Based on natural components.

- Low energy requirement during production.

- Ability to be recycled.

- The material should not include toxic substances.

According to Dr Steve Brown, a research scientist at Australia's Commonwealth Scientific and Industrial Research Organisation CSIRO), building, construction and engineering division, toxic fumes from carpets, paint, furniture and cleaning products can pollute the air inside houses and offices up to seven times the level outside.

In a 1996 study in Adelaide, South Australia, it has been shown that chemical exposure diminishes the reproductive potential of human beings.

Culprits include carpets (especially freshly cleaned carpet), dry- cleaned clothing, particle board and fibreboard walls, solvent based adhesives, sealants, paints, and wood stains used during house construction, deodorisers, vinyl flooring, table surface waxes, insulation, foam couches, and gas heaters.[25]

There are three main categories of material used in construction.

Mineral based material:

Diverse stone, marble, granite, limestone and gravel, sand, glass and plaster.

Metals such as iron, steel, aluminium, zinc, copper, lead and nickel.

Vegetal and animal-based products

Wood and all its derivatives, coco fibre, textiles, oils as base for natural paints, bees wax and wool for carpets.

Chemical materials

Plastic, polyester, synthetic insulation, resins and paints.

In an article published in April 1996 in a Swiss newspaper, Professor Karl Lotz -at the Biberach school of architecture- explained that a mix of building materials should be used in certain proportion to diminish the toxic effects of some of them.

1/3 of hard materials such as concrete and steel.

1/3 of "neutral" materials such as brick and tiles.

1/3 of natural material such as wood, cork, wool.

For each category of material mentioned above there is more specific literature available on the market.

STONE

Stone used in foundations is the best material to transmit tellurian energies to the rest of the structure. By its very nature stone is able to act as an accumulator and amplifier of vibration both cosmic and tellurian.

Traditionally blocks of stone were marked as they were quarried. This natural configuration was respected when the stones were set in place during construction.

Each stone is polarised which means that it has a positive and a negative side. It can be determined with a pendulum, though some experienced stone mason could feel it simply by holding it. The positive side should always be facing outside the construction to enable the energy body of the house to flow in harmony with the environment.

It is best to use stones that have been quarried in the region where the building is to be erected to ensure a certain symbiosis between the site and the house.

Some specific stones used in the construction have special symbolic significance.

The first stone or foundation stone defines the birthday of the building which is sometimes fixed according to astrology. It contains the intention of the builders and there is a celebration when it is placed in the focus point of the nascent dwelling. This centre is defined either by strong tellurian radiation or by an important design feature of the plan.

Another important stone is the threshold stone sometimes flanked on each side by sculptures showing protecting spirits or animals.

The cornerstone has a protecting role and sometimes a niche was carved into it to place a little statue of a god or a saint.

It is interesting that for many sensitive people, stone seems to store the memory of a building, where the history of a space can be imprinted in the very fabric of the walls through the intensity of past events, be they uplifting as in devotional spaces or horrific as in places of murder or torture. This could explain the repulsion or attraction felt in certain buildings as detailed in "The Secret Language of Stone" by Don Robins:

-*Where the mechanism of the interaction between man and stone has been sketched out, we have referred to magnetic encoding networks and trapped electrons and hinted that some binary energising sequence based upon sound pulsing will access a previous coding.*

79

There was also a strong implication that the original trace was put there through some high stress or high emotion event which was itself part of an encoding sequence driven by a pressure pulse through articulated or structured sound, that is through the voicing of the emotions by those involved.... (It is) clear that the decoding sound trigger also had profound effect upon the initiators and audience: they themselves entered into a neuronal or electronic synergism which seemed to give shape and form to the trace buried within stone through the mechanism akin to illusion or hallucination whereby the trace was perceived directly without the mediation of the sensory net, which was overwhelmed by the intensity of the experience."[26]

26 D.Robins (The secret language of stone) Rider London 1988

EARTH

Earth is the most ecological building material; it is abundant, cheap and easy to work. It causes absolutely no recycling problems. It can be used in most climates. It needs well drained foundations and a good wide roof for protection against rain in temperate and humid areas.

When a rammed earth house is built with earth from the site it possesses an added quality of harmony with the environment.

Earth is a material available almost everywhere and requires no special technology to be extracted. It may seem fragile especially in rainy climates, but during the last twenty years

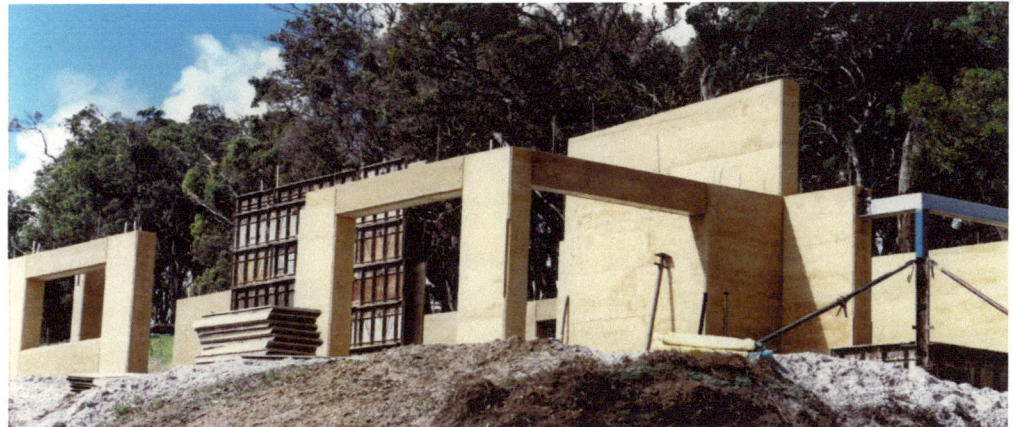

Rammed earth house in Albany WA (JM Gobet)

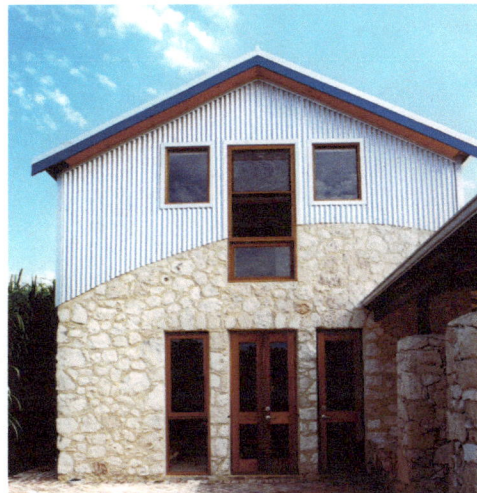

Stone House in Hamilton Hill WA (JM Gobet)

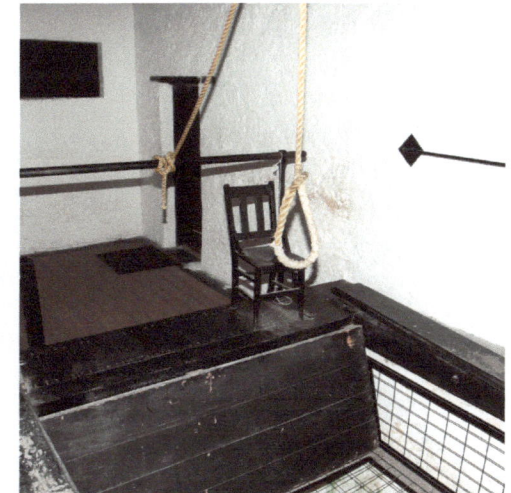

Prison execution room

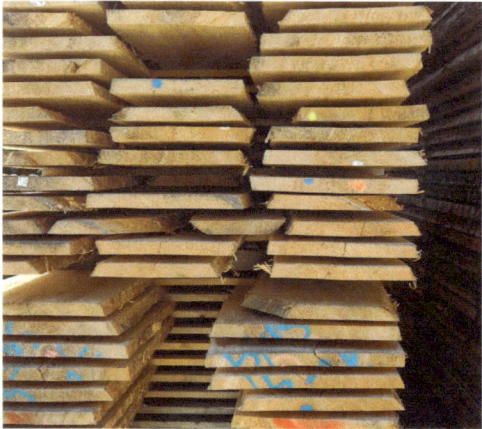

Seasoning wood in Switzerland

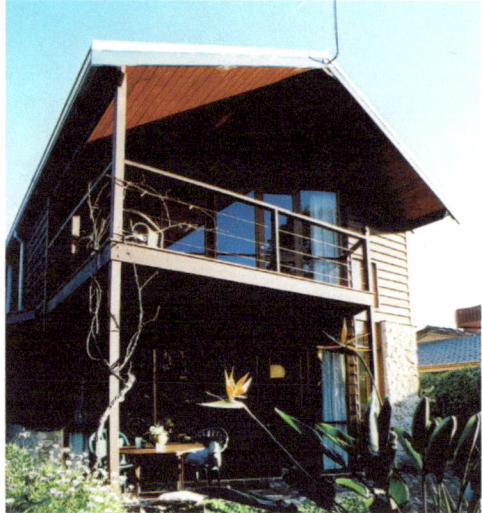

House in Hamilton Hill, Western Australia

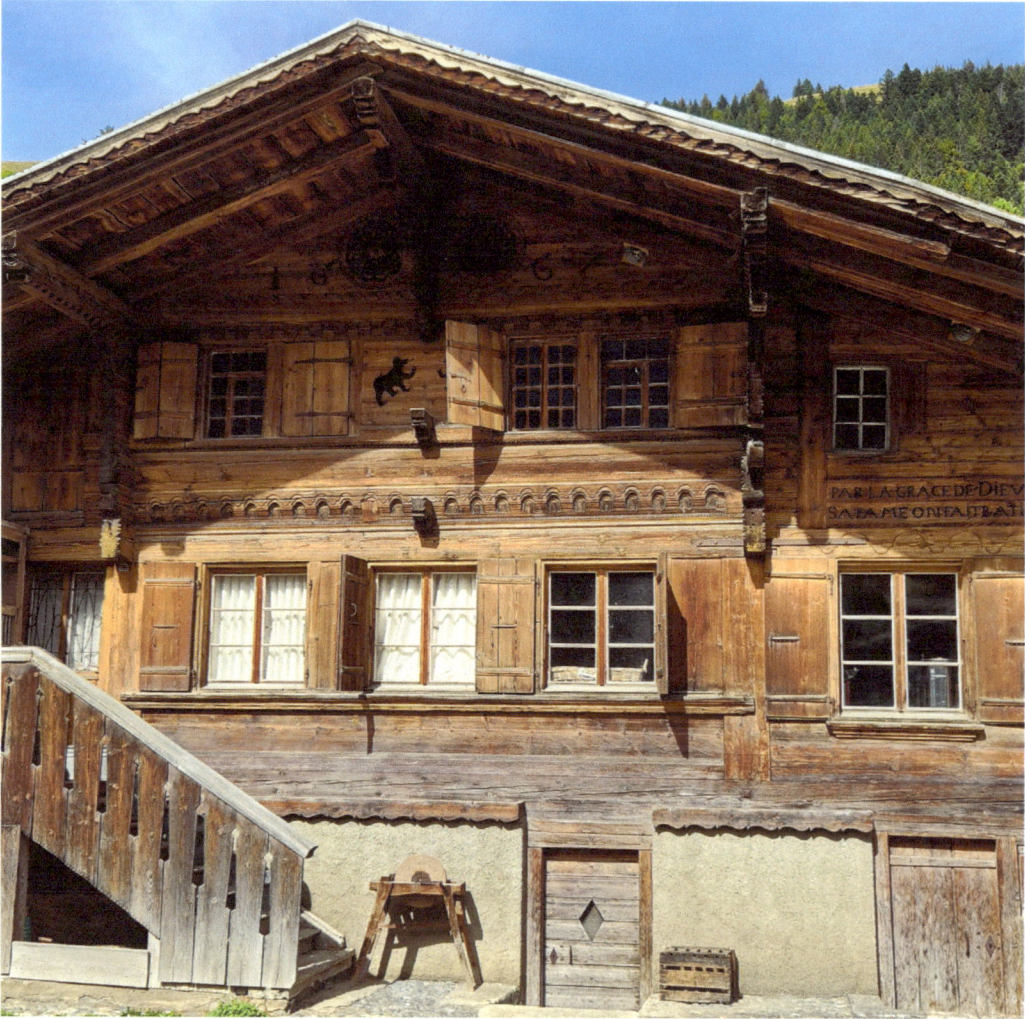

Swiss chalet built in 1667

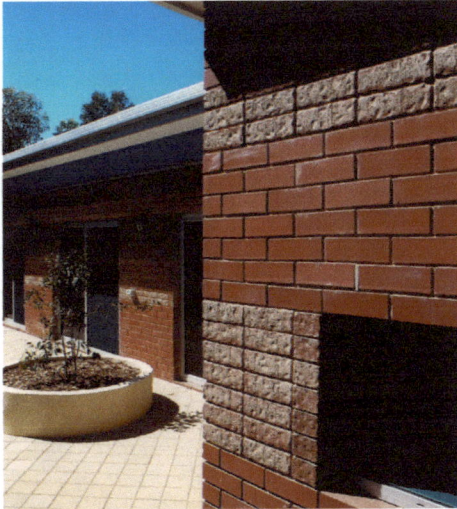

House in Hilton, Western Australia

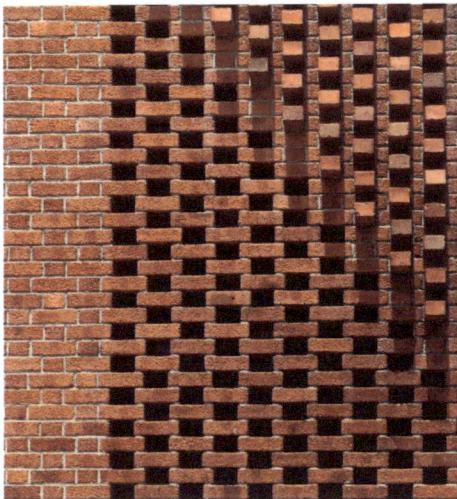

a lot of research has been made to improve the quality of raw earth constructions. Its resistance can be improved by adding straw, reeds or bamboo or by adding cement.

Earth construction is especially comfortable in certain climates due to its great heat inertia. Earth walls regulate the thermal flow and the rate of humidity between the inside and the outside. Another advantage is that earth walls breathe.

Raw earth walls can be built either with rammed earth or with dried earth bricks made on site.

BRICKS

Clay is a natural element; it is one of the best materials from a health point of view. It has great regenerative capacity. It is porous when made into bricks and allows the building to breathe. It is a good regulator of local climatic conditions, warm in winter and cool in summer. It can be used in rammed earth, adobe, hand-made and commercial bricks.

WOOD

In wood, we find almost all the cycles of nature; - the daily cycle of night and day and, -the seasonal cycles of growth and hibernation. We can feel also the four elements -the nourishing cycle of earth and water, the sun's fire for photosynthesis and the air cycle supplying a considerable part of the oxygen we breathe.

These cycles and elements are stored in the very essence of the timber. The fact that it is an organic and living material is its greatest quality. Wherever we find trees we can see timber used for construction. Its structural and insulating qualities make it an ideal building material.

Nowadays economic conditions are controlling the timber industry. The processes of tree felling and timber processing are not in harmony with nature. We are in a vicious circle and we need to return to a more natural and healthy way of working. We compound mistakes and we are left with a product which is often not seasoned properly and has to be treated with toxic substances to avoid further deterioration and attack from insects and fungi.

It is a wonder that nobody asks why some timber constructions in Japan, Russia, Switzerland and Northern Europe are still standing after centuries. I have lived in an Alpine chalet built in 1755 and still in perfect condition. The wood had never been treated or even been painted.

In the Alps of Switzerland a few older carpenters are still inspired by respect for the forest and wood. The trees are felled only during a specific period between December and February, and under the waning moon. Apparently, the phase of the moon influences the property of the cellulosic

27 J.P. Dillenseger
(Habitation et santé)
Editions Dangles

fibres giving them natural insecticide and fungicide properties without need for chemical treatment.

The timber is seasoned for up to 11 years depending on the nature of the wood and its future use. While the wood is being seasoned, it should lie according to its polarity, -the positive corresponding to growth and pointing north.

The polarity of the timber will be respected during construction as well. Each beam, rafter and stud should be carefully positioned according to the original direction of growth of the wood. A tree grows from the earth (negative pole) to the sky (positive pole), thus rafters and studs should always be fixed with their positive pole pointing towards the sky. The beams should have their positive pole pointing towards north or east, to ensure a natural flow of energies between the construction and the biosphere.

The great enemy of timber construction is humidity. The wood should always be kept away from it and should be well ventilated.

As a living material, wood needs to breathe and this fact should be kept in mind when applying surface treatment. Unfortunately, most of the products available on the market nowadays are considered toxic from the point of view of geobiology. Walls, ceilings and floors should not be treated with products which emit toxic gases, seal the wood or allow the accumulation of static electricity.

Interior: It is not always necessary to treat or paint interior wooden surface if they are out of reach, like ceilings for example. If a treatment is necessary one can apply vegetal oils such as linseed. Natural colouring agents can be added (Walnut shell, onion peels). If treated with bees wax the wood will breathe and electrostatic effects will be neutralised. There are now different natural wood treatment and lazures available, which have been developed during the last thirty years, mainly in Germany, France and Switzerland.

Exterior: Traditionally in alpine timber chalets the wood was often protected by being treated with a solution of alkaline salts found in wood ash. The mixture is composed of one unit of ashes for three units of water, boiled for one hour then filtered before use [27]. Nowadays it can be protected with carbolic acid or borax salts.

CONCRETE

In a geobiologically sound construction, the use of reinforced concrete is limited to certain areas such as foundations. In this case, the reinforcing steel rods will be welded or tied together and earthed.

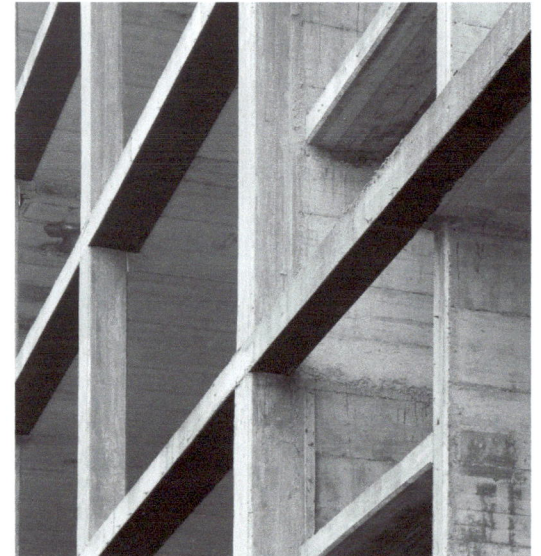

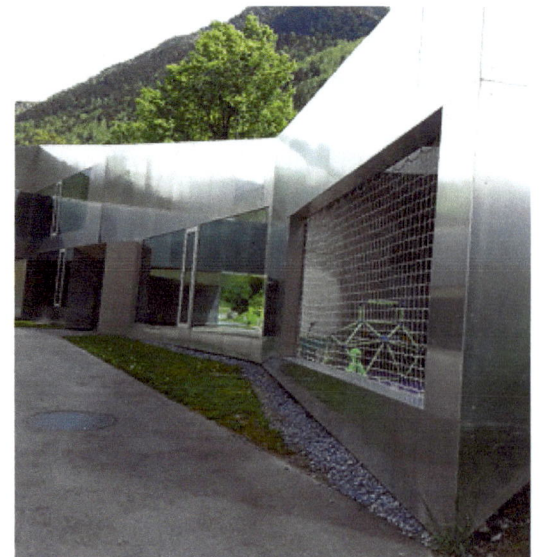

In many cases a concrete slab is poured directly over a bed of compacted sand. The geological nature of the site should be known, in some cases, when building over granitic soil, there might be radon gas emanations. It is then advised to pour the slab over a sealed waterproof membrane to avoid seepage. However, the best solution in such cases is a wooden floor built over a ventilated cavity.

In existing buildings where there are great expanses of concrete, such as walls, slabs and ceilings, one can soften the effects of reinforced concrete with different natural materials.

- Soft wood panelling treated with bees' wax or any biological paint or lazure.

- Cork floor tiles glued with nontoxic biological glues.

- Wool or vegetal fibres carpets and wall coverings. Biological mineral-based paints.

METAL

The metals best suited for bioconstruction are, in decreasing order, copper, zinc, cast iron and galvanised iron. Large surfaces of metal such as roof should be earthed. The same goes for metal columns and the reinforcement of concrete slabs, columns and footings. This is now regular practice in some countries such as Switzerland.

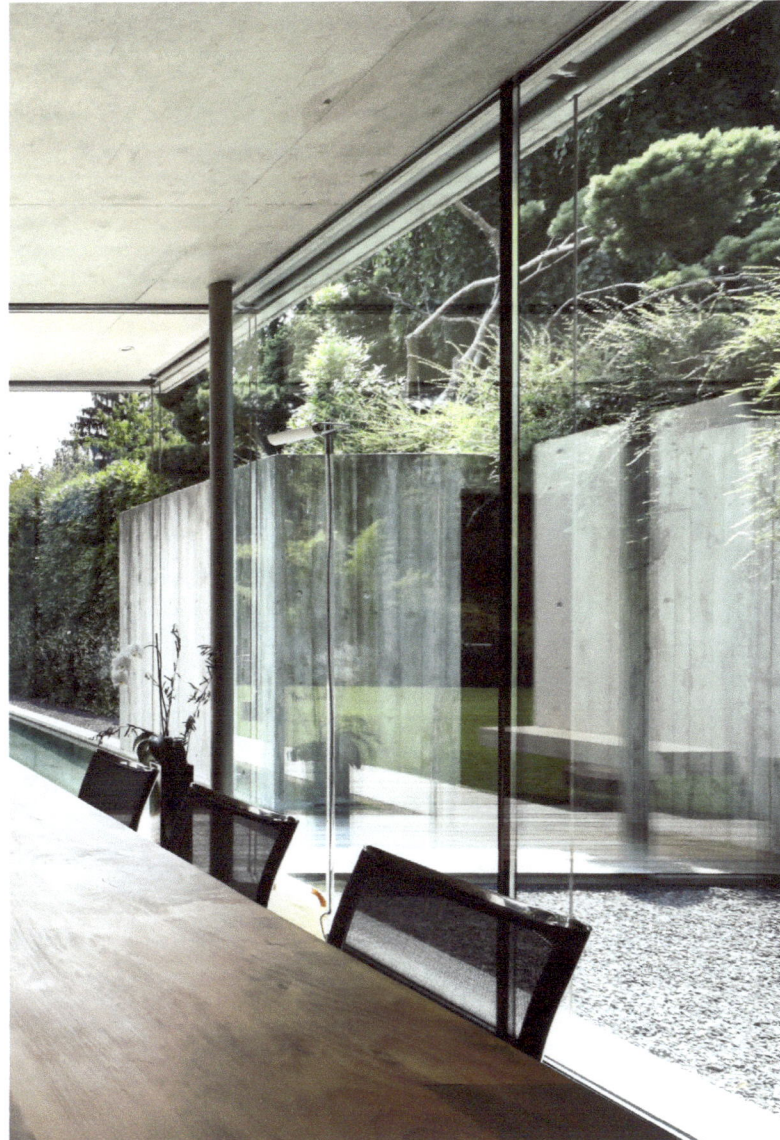

GLASS

There is glass available on the market which lets some U.V. radiation through. This may be good in sun deprived areas like Northern Europe or Canada but would not be suitable in areas such as Australia where U.V. overexposure is a health hazard.

INSULATION

Insulation is a relatively new concept in construction technique. The need for insulating materials grew with the rising cost of petrol in the early 1970s. The Building Industry has offered since a variety of affordable and efficient insulating materials, many of them however are to some degrees not healthy in the long term, both for the inhabitants and the environment in general. Insulation has become essential, first to provide comfort in cold and hot climate but also to reduce the impact of heating and air-conditioning on the climate.

Today we can find on the market different kind of insulation materials:

1. Mineral (Rockwool, Glass wool)

2. Vegetal (Cork, Hemp, Coco fibre)

3. Animal (Sheep wool)

4. Synthetic (Polystyrene boards or beads, Polyurethane)

5. From Recycling (Cellulose, Denim- Cotton)

Mineral

The manufacturing process for rock wool and glass wool is particularly energy hungry and this has to be taken into account for the life cycle of a house. The mineral fibres used to be shaped into batts with formaldehyde based binding agent, nowadays we can find on the market batts made with bio-soluble fibres held together with an acrylic based binding agent. It is necessary to use a steam barrier in conjunction with mineral batts

Animal

Sheep wool has excellent insulating properties, its production and processing have a relatively low impact on the environment.

The batts or rolls are shaped with a binding agent, usually polyester, to ensure that the batts keep their shape and thickness.

Synthetic

Many of the insulating materials used nowadays are produced with fossil fuel. These synthetic products, such as polystyrene and urea foams are not recommended for a healthy house as they produce toxic emanations, especially when burning.

Recycled

*   Cellulose is made with re-used paper, the supply is abundant and it includes the high est content of recycled material of any product on the market. However, it needs to be chemically treated to make it fire resis tant, usually with borax. It is supplied as loose material and it is a good solution to insulate exising houses as it can be injected in the cavity walls. The cavity has to be sealed.

*   Denim insulation is made from scrap and cuttings from jeans factories. It requires little energy to produce and would still be recycla ble at the end of its life as insulation. Unlike cellulose it is less prone to settle thus keeping its insulating capacity.

*   A new generation of ecologically friendly fibre glass batts includes up to 30 percent of recycled glass and none of the petroleum based binding agents, it is a very affordable way to insulate while making sure that the house remains healthy with a product that is non-toxic and respectful of the environment.

Thermal insulation

Special care should be taken to insulate the building against extreme temperature. The roof

85

should be insulated with at least 150mm of insulation, it should not be compressed between the roofing material and the roof battens and/ or the rafters but allowed to expend to its full thickness throughout the roof cavity ensuring that there are no thermal bridges. Stud walls, as well as wooden floors on joists should be insulated with no less than 100mm of insulating material. Windows, French windows and doors should be sealed to avoid too much air exchange.* (These thicknesses are indicative and one should always refer to local building codes).

Acoustic Insulation

The quality of life, especially in a community residing in contiguous houses, will be strongly influenced by the amount of noise transmitted from one dwelling to the other. During the design and construction processes, special care should be taken to insure maximum privacy with the following measures.

- Partition walls should always be doubled, insulated and built up to the roof.

- In houses composed of one floor or more, no slabs should carry from one dwelling to the other.

- Each dwelling should be connected only to its own plumbing. No fittings such as toilets, showers or sinks should be connected to the same downpipe as another dwelling.

- Each dwelling should be fed by its own water supply.

- Each dwelling should be connected to its own hot water system.

- The design of the houses should limit as much as possible the impact of outside sources of noise. Parking areas, roads, playgrounds etc. should be made less disturbing with landscaping, planting and the construction of noise barriers.

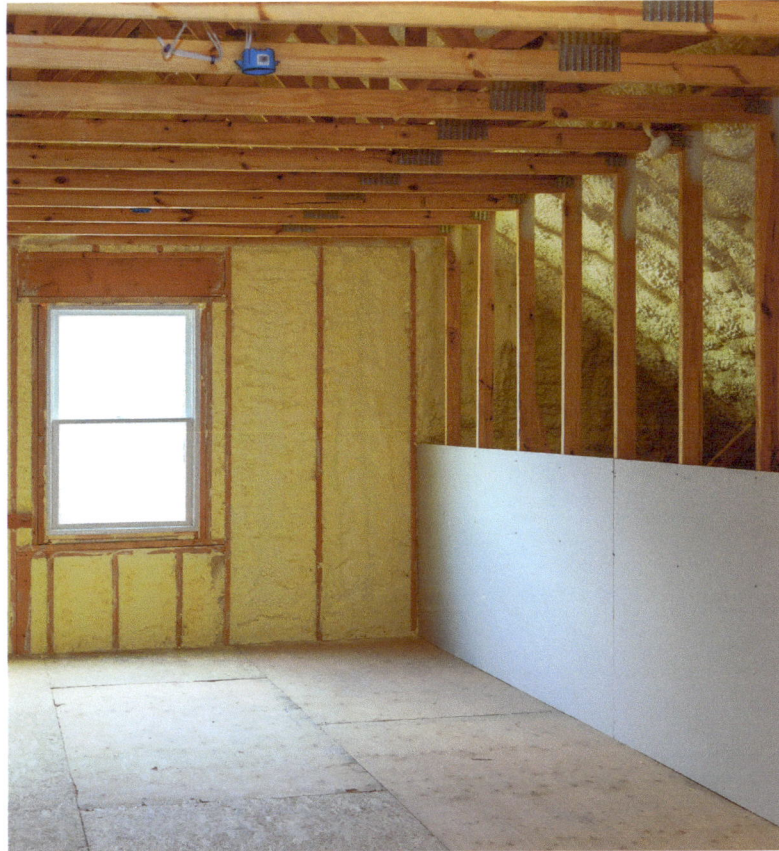

Generally speaking, colour is a power which directly influences the soul. Colour is the keyboard, the eyes are the hammers, the soul is the piano with many strings. The artist is the hand which plays, touching one key or another, to cause vibrations in the soul.

– Wassily Kandinsky (On the spiritual in art) Salomon R. Guggenheim Foundation 1946

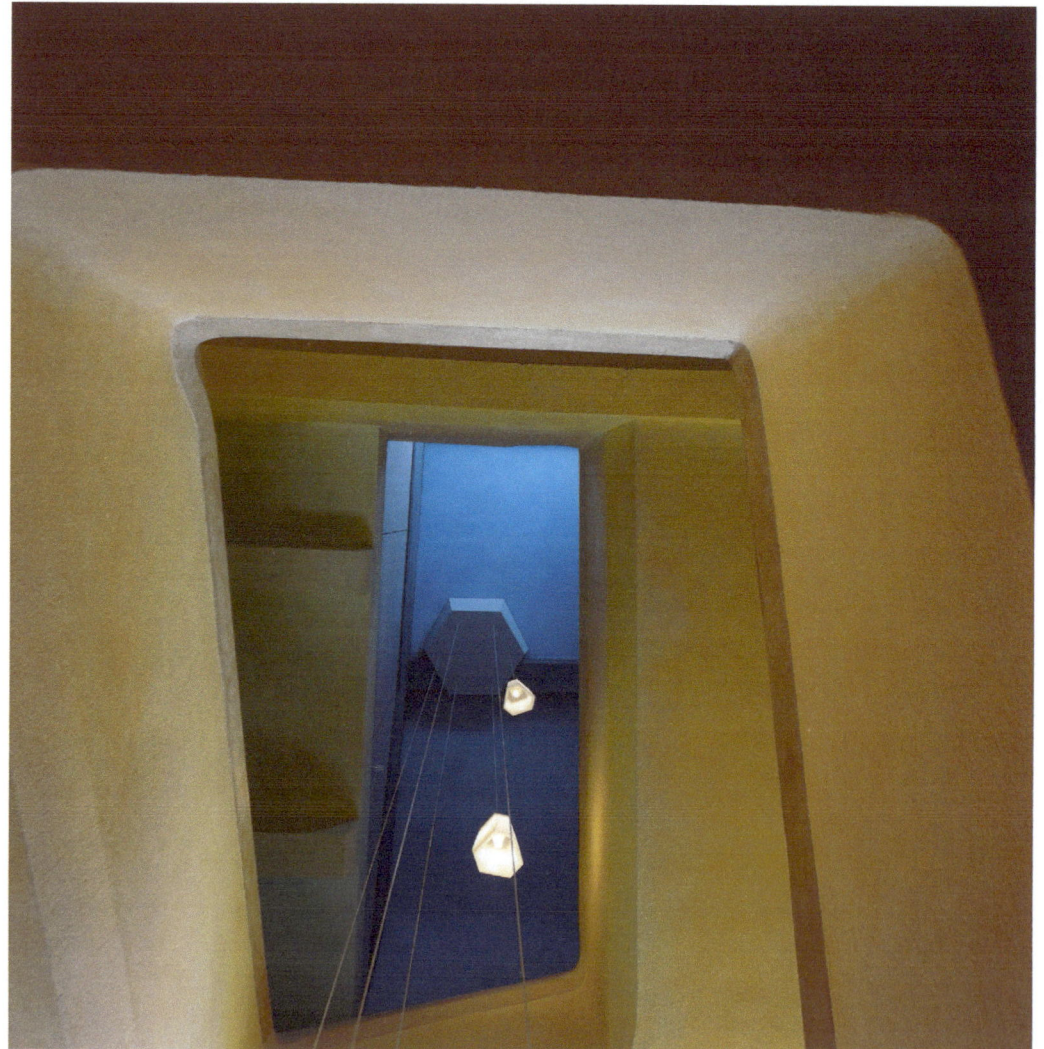

Goetheanum, Switzerland

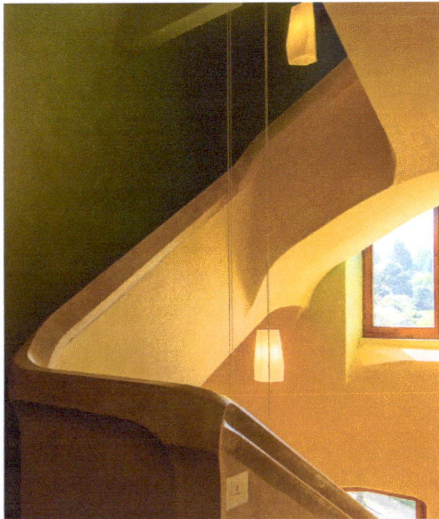

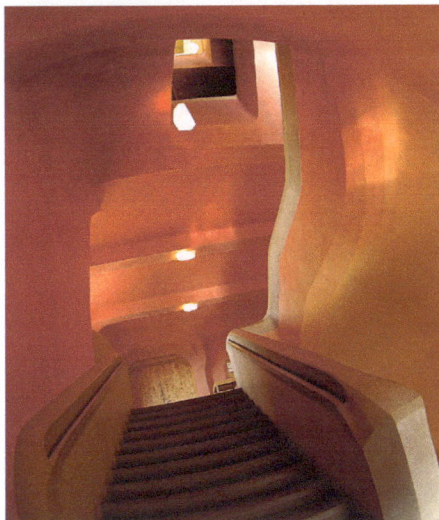

FINISHES

COLOURS AND PAINTS

Since the beginning of time, humans have been fascinated by colours. Some of them, being hard to manufacture have acquired a special status of their own and were reserved for special occasions or special people. The Chinese emperor, for example had the exclusive privilege to wear the colour yellow. For the Roman emperor, it was the colour purple which later became associated with European royalty.

Other colours signified one's characteristics or position in society. Black is almost universally regarded as the colour of mourning and white the colour of purity and virginity.

Chromotherapy

Chromotherapy, the art of healing with colours, assigns to each colour the power to affect our physical, emotional and spiritual wellbeing in a specific way.

Red: stimulates the circulatory system, the blood and warms the spirit, it is expansive and promotes confidence, initiative and courage. Its negative effects are conceit and resentment and should be avoided by people suffering from hysteria and hypertension.

Orange: increases sexual vitality, stimulates the respiratory and digestive systems and brings optimism. It removes repression and inhibition. It broadens the mind and generates more understanding and tolerance. It stimulates the appetite and has a great tonic effect. Its negative aspects are destructiveness and despair.

Yellow: invigorates the nervous system and the digestive system. It also acts on the lymphatic system. It stimulates the intellectual faculties and the logical mind. It promotes self-control Too much of it can bring melancholy and it is not recommended for people suffering from alcoholism or heart problems.

Green: has a calming effect, lowers blood pressure and nervous tension, it helps solving mental or emotional problems. It brings peace and a sense of renewal. It soothes the whole body. Its negative effects are a sense of injustice and grievance.

Blue: induces peace and tranquillity, soothes the nervous system, stimulates the immune system and reduces excessive body heat. It is a contractor and is antiseptic. It helps throat problems and periodic pains. Blue is not recommended for people suffering from rheumatism and hypertension; it could also increase depressive states and generate selfishness.

Indigo: Stimulates parathyroid glands and calms the thyroid gland as well as mental excitement. It purifies the blood and frees the mind of fears. It is related to the senses of sight and hearing. Intolerance might be one of its negative effects.

Purple: closely related to life energy, calms the circulatory system and reduces the effects of anxiety. It stimulates and strengthens spiritual understanding and intuition. Its negative effects are arrogance and fanaticism.

Seeing the effect of different colours on our health, it is wise to use them with care and subtlety. People's need inhabiting the same house can be completely at odds with each other. Even the needs of a particular person can change according to life or seasonal cycles. It is therefore wise to design an environment where the colours of natural materials are predominant. Stronger colours can be used for furniture, rugs, curtains and clothing in a way that leaves the possibility of change when needed.

Paints

Many paints still sold today are synthetic based and toxic. They seal the surfaces on which they are applied and keep the building from breathing thus starting the inevitable cycle of condensation, mould growth and need for more chemical cleaning product to get rid of it.

Furthermore, these paints are composed of highly polluting elements such as synthetic resins, phenols, toluene, xylene, epoxy, ketones, synthetic rubber and heavy metals.

Most of these products are carcinogenic.

Fortunately, more water based, mineral based and even plant base paints are now available and it is easier to choose a product that will not be detrimental to one's health.

Carpet

Wall to wall carpets have become the prevalent way to cover floor areas during the last 50 years.

The availability and relatively low cost of synthetic fibres has made their use common, even in areas where the climate is not suited for them. Traditionally floors were made of earth, tiles or wooden boards, rugs were used seasonally and were easy to clean.

We know that dust mites (acarians) live and die in carpets by the millions. They are a known cause of asthma and of allergic reactions. They usually live in altitudes between 0 and 1000 m above sea level.

Synthetic carpets can emit carcinogenic VOCs (Volatile Organic Compounds) such as formaldeyde and benzene and they increase the level of static electricity in the house.

If a carpet is considered as a floor covering it is best to use natural fibres and to clean them regularly. There exists now on the market vacuum cleaners equipped with a high temperature dry steam jet which cleans, kills and gets rid of dust mites without the inconvenience of chemical products.

Vinyl

Vinyl is very prevalent in the building industry due to its affordability. It is a petroleum-based material made from polyvinyl chloride (PVC) resins with plasticisers, pigment and fillers. Safety standards have improved in the last ten years but one must be aware of Vinyl products made with recycled plastics manufactured when building regulations were less stringent, the older plastics are known to contain toxic components. In ancillary areas such as a laundry or a toilet a vinyl floor finish could be an acceptable compromise, not so in a living space or a bedroom.

Linoleum

Linoleum is a healthy alternative to Vinyl, it is made with natural organic components such as linseed oil, marble, cork or wood dust and pine resin, it possesses natural bactericidal properties, it is very long lasting and fairly easy to maintain.

89

Timber

When a timber floor is ordered, one should always make sure it is produced with certified legally harvested wood. A solid timber floor rejoices the soul, it is pleasing to the eye and soft to the touch. It should be treated with natural product, from bees wax to vegetal oils and essences, it will thus keep its ability to breathe.

Tiles

Ceramic tiles and terra-cotta tiles are a durable and healthy material, they are easy to produce and maintain. In hot and dry climates, they feel cooler than carpet. In winter, it is easy to add a few rugs to improve the room's comfort.

Terrazzo

Terrazzo is an in-situ concrete pour with addition of coloured sand, gravel and small stones which is then machine polished. It is more expensive than tiles but it can be personalised to the taste of the owner. It is very long lasting and easy to maintain.

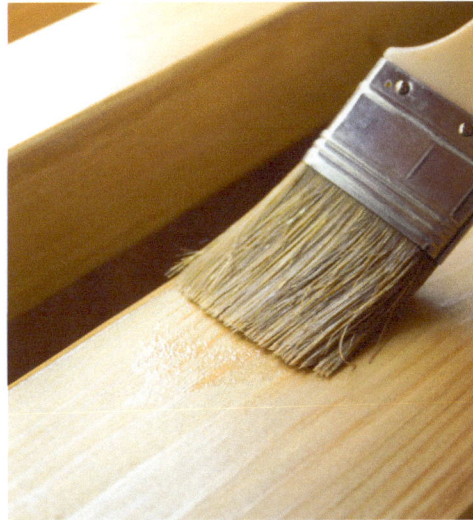

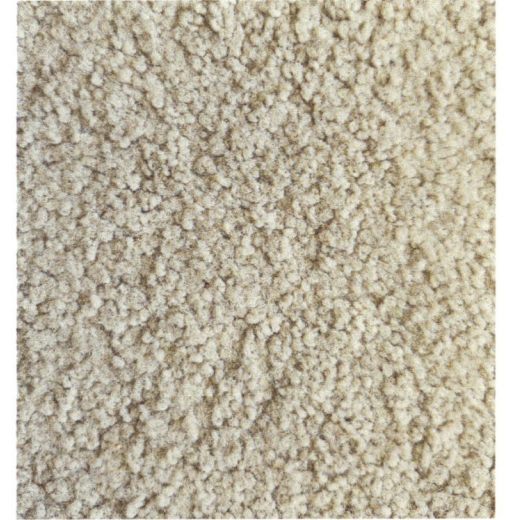

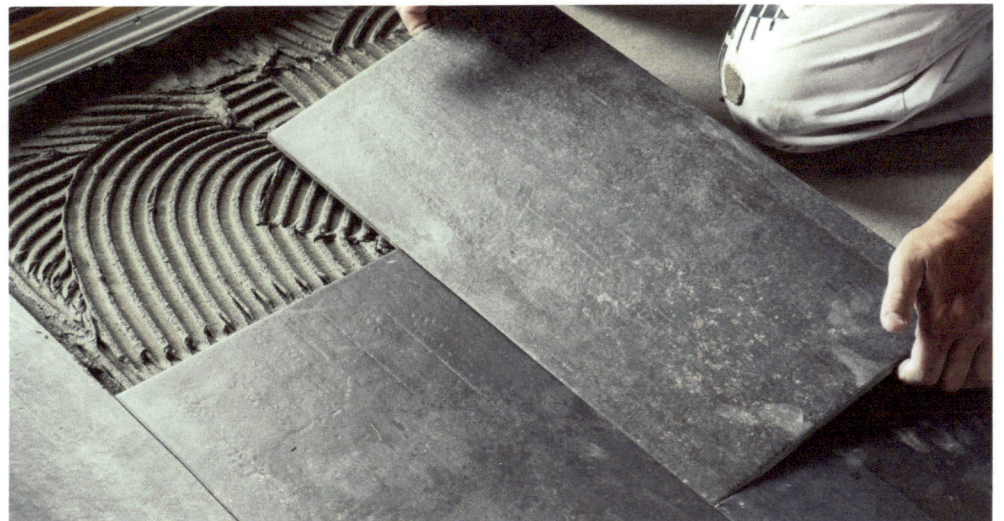

07 /
Energy

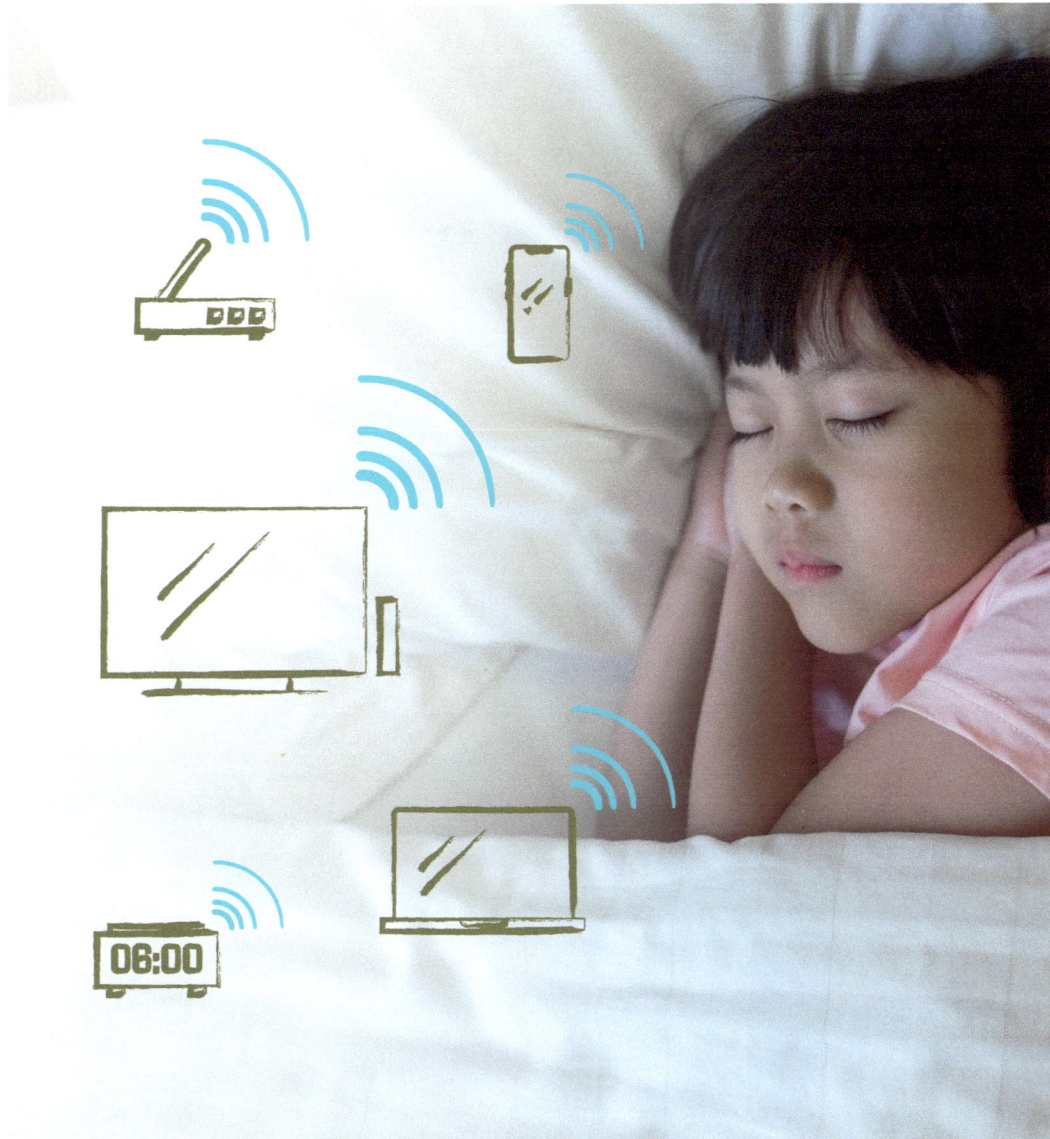

ELECTRICITY

ELECTRICITY ELECTROMAGNETIC POLLUTION

During the last 100 years the use of electricity, a relatively new discovery, has increased considerably. It has dramatically changed the natural electromagnetic field in which we evolved as organisms.

It is now in every part of our environment. In our cities there are power plants, power lines and transformers. In our homes electricity is now everywhere from the kitchen to the bedroom. Every electrical installation and every appliance whether switched on or not has an electrical field. This field reacts differently depending on its charge, either positive or negative.

Electric fields are "natural" when generated by solar activity, air movement, storms and cosmic radiation producing ionisation of the air.

They are "artificial" when produced by man-made activities.

The artificial electric fields have become by far the most important in our living and working place.

Every variation of the electrical field can have an effect on our organism. This, added to other environmental factors such as air and noise

28 The Influence
of Electromagnetic
Pollution
on Living Organisms:
Historical Trends and
Forecasting Changes
(Grzegorz Redlarski et
al.) BioMed Research
International Volume
2015 Article 234098

29 Article in DW
27.01.2004

pollution and stress, can cause an imbalance resulting in discomfort and even disease. Some of the symptoms are insomnia and high blood pressure.

A hundred years ago, electricity was connected to wood, stone or brick houses to light up a few 40-watt bulbs.

Nowadays electricity is connected to houses built with materials such as reinforced concrete, metal frames and synthetic materials to power an extensive range of electrical appliances such as fridges, stoves, TVs, washing machines, dryers, dishwashers, juicers and computers and a host of other "time-saving" devices. We live within a web of electric wiring.

In 1986, after studying 550 houses in Denver - Colorado, David Savitz concluded that the risk of cancer is increased by 50 per cent in the vicinity of high-voltage power lines.

In another study made in 1979 of 963 houses in the same area his colleagues Nancy Wertheimer and Ed Leeper noticed an increase of 100 per cent in the incidence of cancer and leukaemia in children living near high power lines.

Animals can also be strongly affected by electromagnetic fields. According to Dr Andrew Marino and Robert Becker of the New York Veteran Hospital they can diminish the fertility

of rats. *"Other examination results reported and published in the literature were carried out among Swiss railway workers and suggested endocrine system disorders in many cases. The side effects were observed after a 5- day exposure to magnetic fields, where the field frequency was 16.7 Hz. A decreased excretion of melatonin related compounds in the urine was also observed in the case of those workers, who were exposed to magnetic fields of frequencies of 60 Hz. These changes were observed after the second day of their working week."*[28]

In 1989, Electricity of France (EDF) and the companies supplying electricity in Ontario and Quebec published the results of a study of 40,000 French and Canadian people. According to this study electric installation and distribution inside the home and electric appliances could cause more health problems than high power lines.

Beside the extremely low frequencies (ELF) generated by the distribution of electricity, electromagnetic pollution is also caused by radio frequencies and microwaves which can induce a "cooking effect".

After the Second World War, many radar operators died because of internal burns after having been exposed for too long and being too close to the source of radiation without protection.

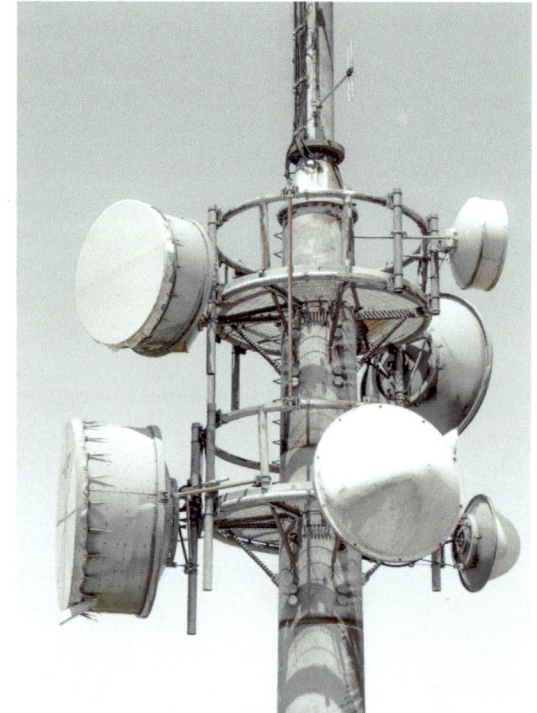

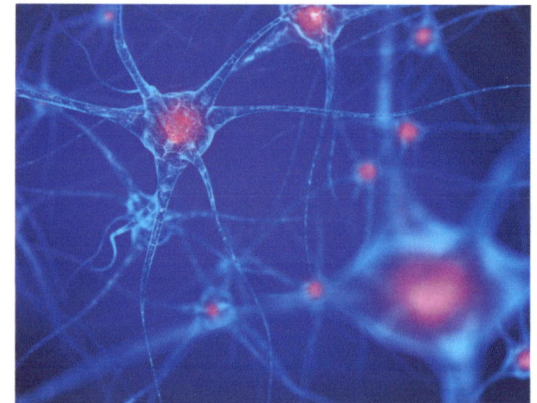

93

30 The Australian
(10 May 1996)

31 Mark Balfour (The
sign of the Serpent,
Key to Creative Physics)
Prism Press

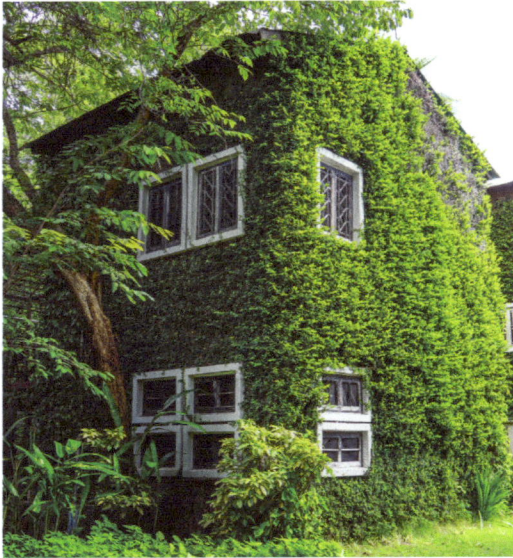

Ivy growing on elevations facing power line will help earth the electromagnetic field and shield the occupants

"A United States Court in El Paso, Texas, on Monday agreed to hear a case brought on by German Bundeswehr soldiers suffering from leukemia or testicular cancer who claim they contracted their illness after exposure to radar equipment made by American defense contractors like Raytheon, Lucent Technologies and ITT Industries. [29]

According to Dr Bruce Hocking, a consultant in occupational medicine and former chief medical officer for Telecom Australia, data analysed from the New South Wales Cancer Registry on cancer incidence between 1972 and 1990 and found 100 cases of childhood leukaemia and just under 40 deaths. The children were living in three Sydney districts close to television towers have a 60 per cent higher rate of childhood leukaemia than children in adjacent areas. [30]

Being in the near field of a transmitter of radio frequency radiation, including microwave radiation for sustained periods of time is hazardous to human health and can promote the development of some types of cancer.

The human body is in fact a microcosm, a subtle interplay of energies, held together in a state of harmony by the forces of attraction and repulsion usually called electromagnetism.

"Evidence now exists that the essential view of life is characterised not by chemical reactions but by information carrying electromagnetic fields. Within this framework, explanation of all biological processes, for example health, ageing, cancer, communication, biological rhythms, regulation and biochemical control, may be found." (Announcement in 1989 from the Institute of Physics, Chinese Academy of Sciences- Beijing)

Cells as "conscious living entities" are highly sensitive to a wide range of electromagnetic fields, either manmade or arising from neighbouring electromagnetic activity in the biophysical system.

Nutritional shortcomings, environmental discord, ultraviolet irradiation, drug abuse, sustained adverse mental or emotional strain, repression of creative desires, geopathic stress and genetic factors all contribute to field disturbance, cell vulnerability as well as immune system deficiency. Freedom from disease ultimately relies on one's ability to maintain equilibrium between a natural vibratory state and abnormal influences that may disrupt it. [31]

During the course of my practice as an architect I have come across many cases of acute reaction to electromagnetic pollution. These people had to move to the countryside where the density of power lines and phone transmission towers was minimal. It seems that there is an added individual component in how one is reacting to electromagnetic pollution, just as there is a wide variation within a population as to how an individual reacts to pollen or any other potentially allergenic substances.

The aim of geobiological design is to provide an environment where the risk of electromagnetic pollution is minimised.

Outside the house

When choosing a site or a house one should avoid high-power lines, transformers or power plants.

Power lines have different effects on the environment; electromagnetic and electrostatic effects, production of ozone and nitrogen oxides, and radio wave emissions. They can also produce an irritating humming noise.

According to Dr Henry Quinquandon a 60,000-volt power line will have a disturbing effect on the environment as far as 200 metres away.

A study by Karl Lotz show that a transformer will affect the environment up to seven meters on the north side and up to 25 meters on the south side, the difference being caused by the movement of the geomagnetic field.

In case of high electromagnetic pollution, a copper net can be placed between the source of pollution and the house, it should be earthed. Ivy or other creepers growing on walls, as well as pine trees planted between houses and power lines are known to earth disturbing electromagnetic fields.

Metal roofs, gutters or any other metal structure, if earthed properly can be of great help in diminishing the impact of a nearby power line.

Certain architectural elements such as towers and oriels capped with metal roofs or metal ornament such as weathervanes or spikes act as antennae. If they are not earthed properly (on the north side) they will be charged with static electricity. The same applies to TV antennae; they should be earthed as well and never be placed over a bedroom.

Inside the house

To illustrate the danger of electromagnetic pollution inside a home, let us take the worst possible example. Let us assume Mr. X is living near a power line, on the first floor of a house built with a reinforced concrete slab whose metal reinforcement is not earthed. The bedroom is situated over the garage, over the heavy metallic mass of the car, disturbing the natural geomagnetic field. The bedroom is a particularly sensitive area; this is where we lie for up to eight hours straight in the same spot, defenceless, while our body tries to regenerate. Let us now assume Mr. X sleeps in a metal bed on a mattress with metal coils and he uses an electric blanket always plugged in whether in use or not. There are power points near the head of the bed, an electric alarm clock, a stereo and even a television. The room is lined with wall-to-wall synthetic carpet. Mr. X does not sleep well, he suffers from recurrent migraines. He drinks herbal tea in the evening and worries about his diet, but nothing really

helps. He only feels good when he goes in the country for a camping trip, though it would be so simple to change his environment.

Some useful precautions can be taken to avoid or minimise the impact of electromagnetic pollution.

- Power lines should be laid underground.

- Use shielded cables for the distribution.

- Avoid cables looping around the rooms. It is preferable to distribute the electricity in a herringbone or star pattern.

- Use switches to turn the electricity off at the power point at certain times in certain areas, for example the bedroom at night.

- The most important aspect is to have the installation well earthed. In a geobiologically designed house the resistance should not be above 10-15 ohms.

- Avoid electrical appliances in the bedroom (TV, stereo, telephone) hi fi speakers generate an electromagnetic field.

- Avoid placing a bed or a workstation near the meter box.

- Avoid material that will be electrostatically charged such as synthetic carpet, vinyl wallpapers, plastic or metal furniture, wide areas of metal and synthetic insulation materials.

- Avoid bedrooms over garages or parking.

GROUNDING

Even when living in areas affected by electromagnetic pollution it is possible to diminish its impact by grounding oneself. Walking barefoot in dew covered grass or on the beach will quickly restore the body's natural balance.

EARTHING TECHNIQUES

The way the electrical installation is earthed is considered very important in geobiology, and it has a direct influence on the quality of the habitat. It should be especially made according to geobiological guidelines. The electrode should be situated outside the perimeter of the construction and preferably on the northern side, on a neutral zone. The earth electrode is a vital element of the house, without it, it can be saturated with electrical pollution.

The resistance of the electrode depends on its size, shape, and the resistance of the ground in which it is set.

Soil resistance:

The electrode's resistance is proportional to the resistance of the ground in which it is buried.

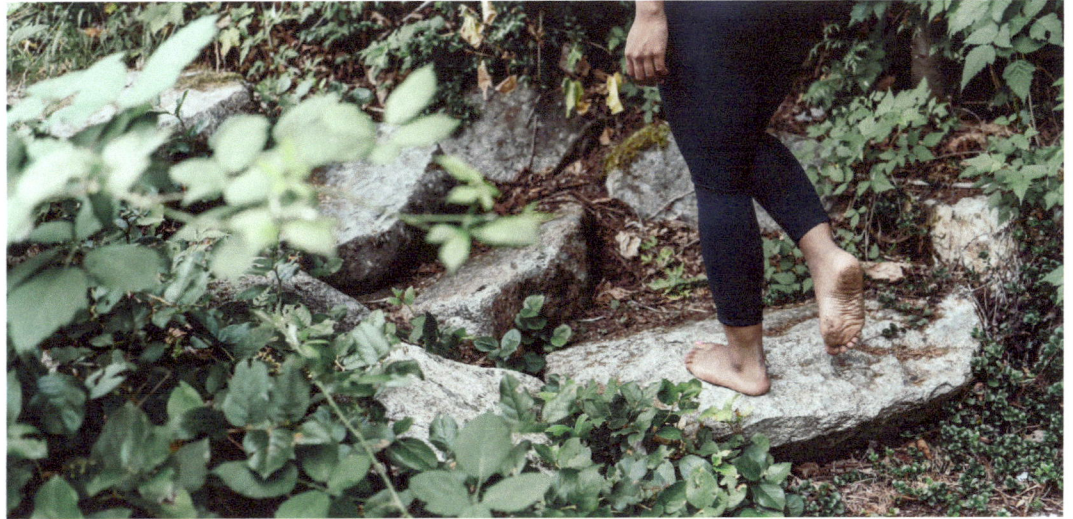

The resistance of the ground is measured in ohms per metre and is defined as the resistance of a volume of soil of one cubic metre.

It can vary strongly from one area to another depending on the nature of the ground, the size of the particles, how well compacted they are and the level of humidity. The resistance can vary from 20 ohms for a humid and dense soil to a few thousand ohms for dry granitic rock formations.

In any given area, the ground can be heterogeneous, which means that is composed of different layers of materials, vertically as well as horizontally. The resistance of a particular soil is also affected by seasonal variations, due to draught or frost. It is then advisable to bury the electrode more than one metre below the surface.

If the soil is composed mainly of gravel and big stones it will not earth the electricity well at all. Firstly, it will not have the ability to retain moisture and secondly it will not allow good contact with the electrode. In such a case, it is advisable to surround the electrode with fine earth or sand or any other good conducting material.

Apart from a few materials such as iron ore, most rocks have a very high resistance, which is only reduced by humidity.

Electrodes:

In a geobiologically sound construction, the resistance of the earth should not exceed 10 ohms. It can be achieved when special care is taken when installing the electrode.

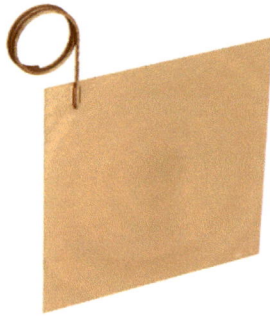

Metal plate electrode

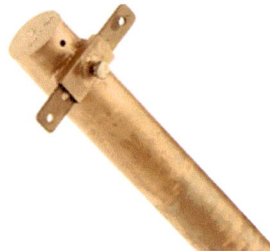

Vertical electrode rod

As much as possible the electrode should be buried lower than the level of constant humidity, and an increase of resistance due to corrosion needs to be considered. The determining factors diminishing the resistance of the electrode are its shape and dimension.

There are three different types of electrodes.

- Horizontal electrodes: Copper cables at least 25mm². Aluminium electrode minimum section 35mm² protected with lead. Steel cables minimum section 95mm². These electrodes can be either buried in a trench all around the foundations or in special trenches one meter deep filled with earth which should be kept humid.

- Metal plates: Metal plates measuring 0.5m x 1m or 1m x 1m buried vertically at a depth of one metre at their centre. They should be 2mm thick if made from copper or 3mm if made from galvanised steel.

- Vertical electrodes: Galvanised steel tubes minimum 25mm diameter. Extruded steel profiles 60mm side.

Copper or galvanised steel bars minimum 15mm diameter. They should be long enough to reach the level of constant humidity and below frost level.

SOLAR ENERGY

The technology of solar energy capture and storage has come a long way in the last 20 years. We are on the verge of being able to devote the entire external skin of a house to the capture of solar energy as new photovoltaic roof tiles and even photovoltaic paints are being developed. The means of storing it has also become much better and cheaper.

SOLAR PASSIVE ARCHITECTURE

Vernacular architecture fulfilled most of the criteria of what is now known as solar passive architecture. It relied on local skills and local materials to provide dwellings best suited to the local climate, it generated a homogeneous urban fabric without diminishing the individual beauty and uniqueness of each house. We can still be delighted by walking through old towns in Europe, Asia or Africa. Every climate and geographic location offer exquisite architectural ways to provide comfort and security.

With the advent of the XXth century, cooling and heating relied more and more on fossil fuel energy and traditional building techniques gave way to mass production of cheap construction materials.

As we have become more aware of our impact on the environment, traditional know-how combined

97

with the latest building technology can provide new solution for sustainable and environmentally friendly housing.

WIND ENERGY

It is now possible to access small vertical wind turbines to generate electricity on residential sites. The required condition is a steady laminar wind flow, usually prevalent in coastal areas and the open countryside. Urban areas, rough terrain and heavily wooded areas do not lend themselves to wind generated power as turbulence makes it difficult for the wind turbine to operate at its full potential.

ENERGY SAVINGS

Through aware and competent design, the building will consume considerably less energy than the average traditional house and moreover will be improved by the choice of energy saving appliances.

- Energy efficient fridges, washing machines and dishwashers.

- Solar hot water systems.

- Demand switches.

- Good insulation of roofs and walls.

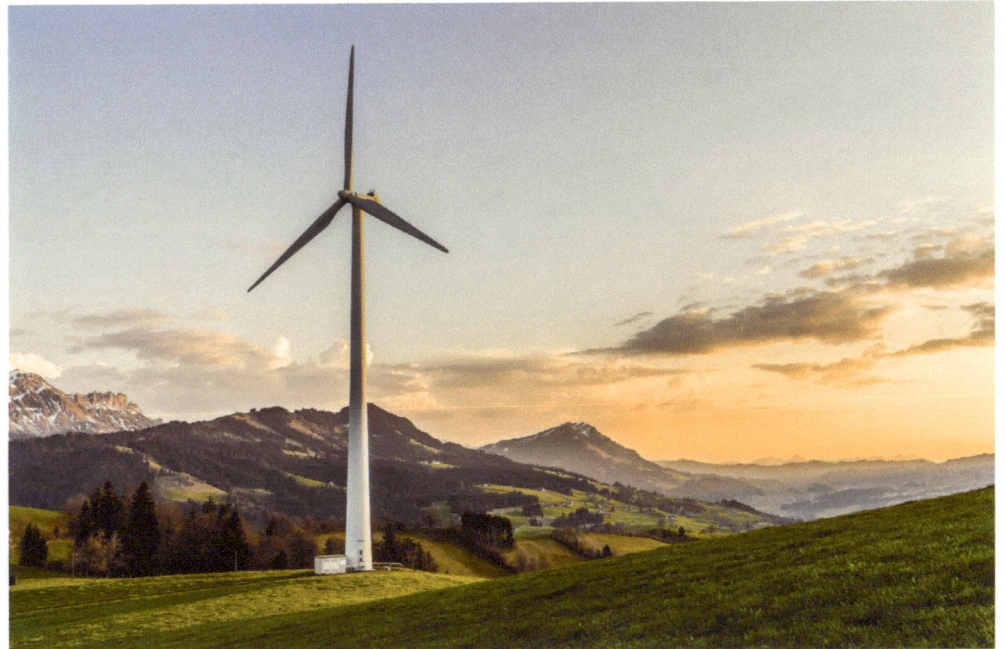

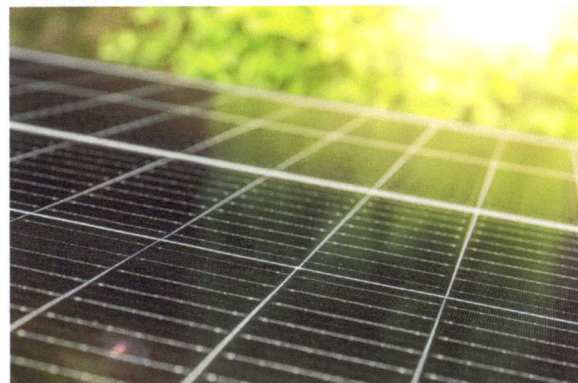

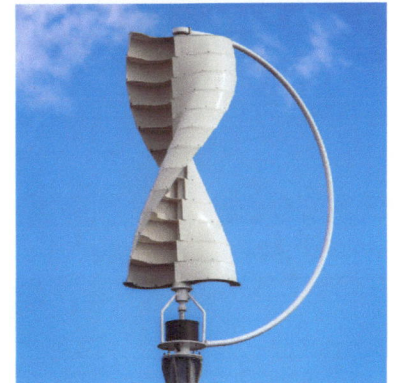

08 /
Water

99

"We must pay respect to water, and feel love and gratitude, and receive vibrations with a positive attitude. Then water changes, you change, and I change. Because both you and I are water."

– Masaru Emoto, The True Power of Water

To the Aborigines of the north west of Australia, water is the means through which spirit incarnates on Earth. It is not merely essential to the development of organic life but is primarily a support for consciousness.

We find a similar view in the work of the Austrian naturalist Johan Grander who considered that water has a memory and can carry information between different systems including living organisms. Homeopathic medicine is also based on water's memory and its ability to transfer information.

It is the only substance found in all three states of matter at ordinary temperatures, as a solid when crystallised as ice, as a liquid in its most common state and as a gas when reduced to vapour.

Due to its ability to dissolve elements, pure water is not usually found in nature. It carries

microorganisms and micro particles of mineral elements.

Water is one of the best-known ionising agents, ionisation being the process by which atoms and molecules can be electrically charged

The spectrographic study of water vapour reveals a structure similar to an isosceles triangle, its summit being an atom of oxygen and its two lower angles being two atoms of hydrogen. Water is thus a polarised molecule and it is electromagnetically charged. It could be compared to a small magnet.

In nature, water never moves in a straight line, it meanders through the landscape; it naturally tends to assume round and spherical shapes, whether through waves or whirlpools. The whirling action of water will ionise it and the direction of the whirling whether to the left or right, will determine the negative or the positive charge.

The movement of water against the sides of an underground stream or against a riverbank generates electromagnetism. It is this slight difference of potential which, according to the French physicist Yves Roccard, enables the dowser to find water.

Water is not merely an element, it is a process, an ongoing cycle of evaporation, crystallisation and precipitation. When we intervene and

disturb this harmonious cycle -by polluting the air where water evaporates, the earth through which it filters, and by polluting water itself

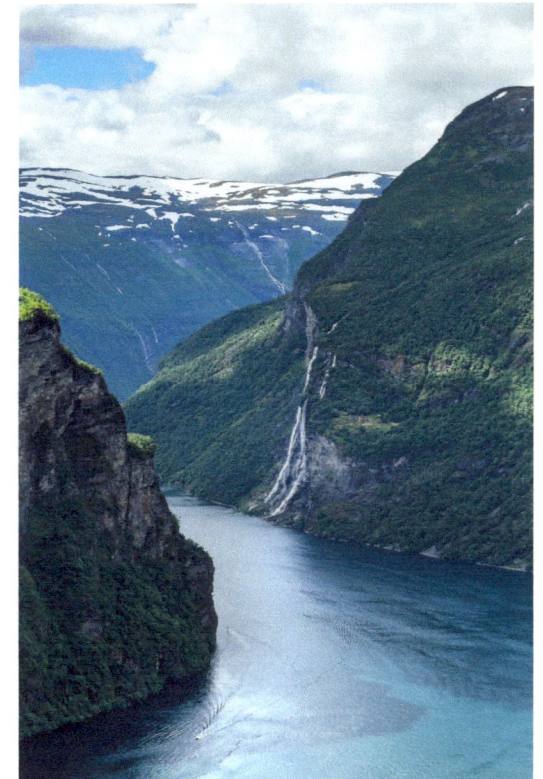

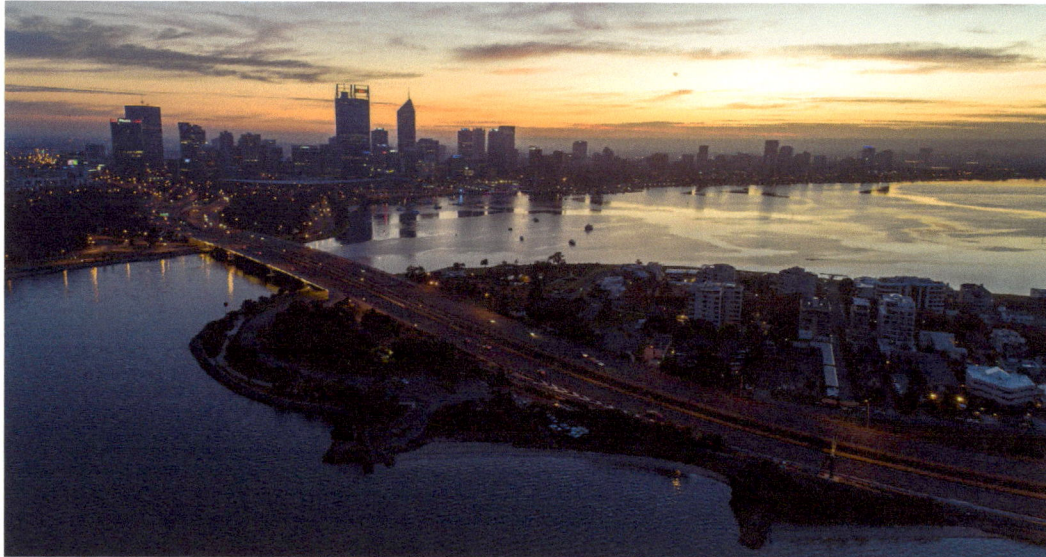

with domestic and industrial effluents- it is not enough to take care of the chemical treatment of water but it is essential to revitalise it, to infuse it with life.

WATER IN THE LANDSCAPE

Every human settlement has developed in the vicinity of water. In addition, as a prerequisite for survival, it has become a symbol of the gift of life. Even though technology has enabled us to transport water far from its source, the presence of water on a given site is a great asset and can dramatically modify the quality of the environment.

- As a visual element, reflecting the surrounding nature.

- As sound, running water or waterfalls have a soothing effect.

- As a natural generator of negative ions, it will increase the sense of wellbeing in the area. This is especially true in the hot and arid climates.

- As a habitat for a variety of animal species it will increase the biodiversity of the site.

WATER CONSERVATION

In an environmentally conscious project, a water saving policy should be implemented at the design stage.

Collecting rain and storm water from the roofs and the roads is the first step in keeping the water on the site as long as possible. The advantages of this approach are the availability of this water to be used on the site and to make water more prominent in the planning of the landscape.

The natural slope of a site offers the opportunity of other means to keep and store water on the site by planting along banks, while dams, ponds and small waterfalls are natural negative ion generators, Rocks should be placed in streams to create flowing forms, eddies and increase the sound of running water. Wetlands should be restored and water catchment areas kept free from construction. Both these areas are fragile ecosystems and essential for the quality of the water cycle.

The landscape and gardens should be planted with local species adapted to the average yearly rainfall thus necessitating little watering.

- Each fitting and appliance should be assessed on its ability to save water.

- Low flush or dual flush toilets should be installed.

- Compost toilets in rural communities should be encouraged.

- Water saving shower heads should be installed in all bathrooms.

- Flow control aerator or water saving taps should be systematically used.

- Appliances such as washing machines and dishwashers should be assessed on their water consumption performance.

- Grey water recycling systems should be installed. Grey water recycling involves the collection of bath and shower water. This water is filtered and then reused for watering the garden or flushing the toilet. Knowing that most of our drinking quality water is used to flush toilets makes a considerable saving.

- Rainwater should be collected and stored.

- Whenever possible, especially in rural communities, special care should be taken to ensure that water is treated, revitalised and restored to its pristine purity before leaving the property.

WATER TREATMENT

Most modern cities are taking care of water treatment and every house is usually connected to the system.

Industrial size water treatment plants use a combination of physical and chemical processes to treat

GREYWATER SOURCES

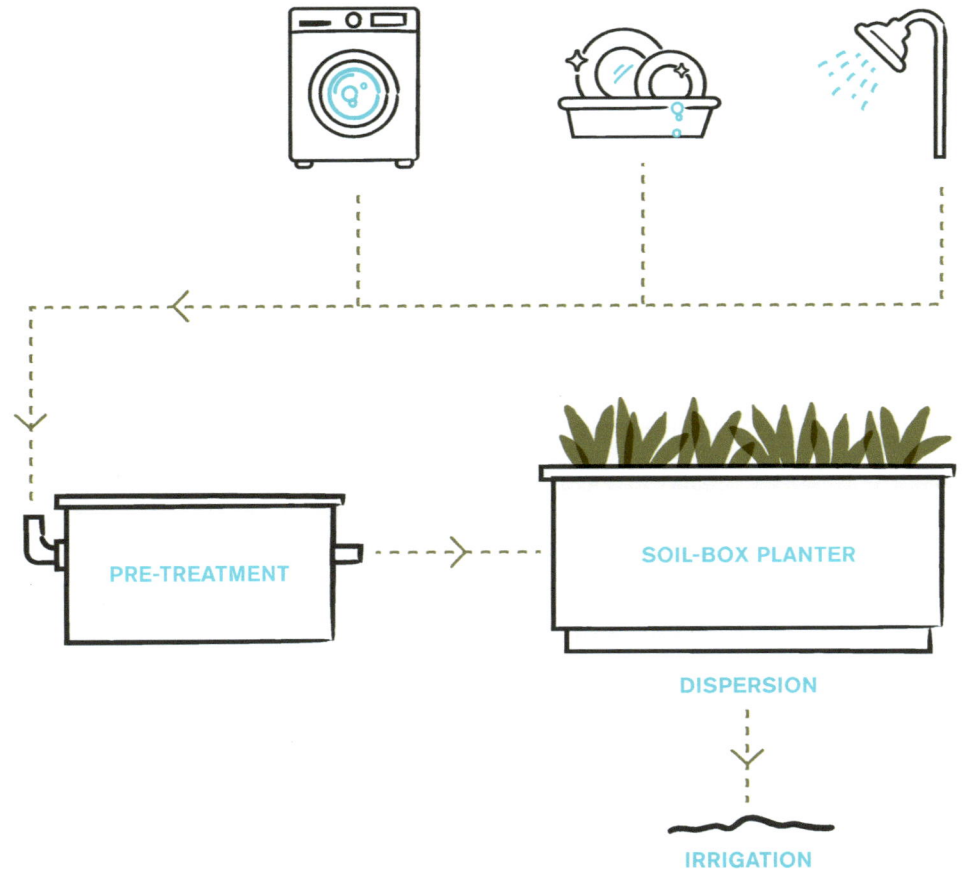

PRE-TREATMENT

SOIL-BOX PLANTER

DISPERSION

IRRIGATION

102

32 The water wizard (Viktor Schauberger- Callum Coats) Gateway

"The majority believes that everything hard to comprehend must be very profound. This is incorrect. What is hard to understand is what is immature, unclear and often false. The highest wisdom is simple and passes through the brain directly into the heart."

– Viktor Schauberger

dirty waters, such as sedimentation, filtration and chlorination. But biological water treatment systems are now becoming more common, even in large scale treatment plants.

Biological water treatment uses a variety of microorganisms and bacteria to digest organic matter into simpler substances. Many domestic size systems are now available.

WATER REVITALISATION

There are three facets to evaluate the water quality:

- The chemical constituents.

- The organic aspect including contamination by diverse pollutants.

- The "energetic" quality of water.

The first two aspects are usually taken care of in developed societies where we have access to clean water free of pathogens.

Many of us are not satisfied with our chlorinated tap water, we buy bottled "spring" water or we install filtration systems in order to drink the all elusive "life giving" fresh water we desperately need.

This is because even without being fully conscious of it, we instinctively know and feel the difference between tap water that feels lifeless and fresh spring water which refreshes and rejuvenates.

Water which has become drinkable through industrial treatment will be clear and sterile but would have lost all the qualities that fresh water from a mountain stream possesses following its transit through the landscape. After this natural cycle it will be oxygenated, vivified and acquire a life-giving energy.

According to Viktor Schauberger[32], there are many kinds of water and H_2O in its pure chemical state is merely its juvenile and sterile form which is poisonous to living things as in the long term it would leach out all minerals.

For water to mature and reach its full life-giving potential it needs to pass through its natural cycle of precipitation, soaking into the landscape, sinking into layers of rocks and sediments to be mineralised and finally surge from a spring and roll over cascades, rocks and riverbeds, creating eddies and vortices. Water is not a passive element; it inscribes its passage with its pulsating inner rhythms and re-shapes the landscape.

These life-giving eddies and vortices are key to the water energising process, they have been studied and reproduced in the "flow forms" designed by John Wilkes in the 1970s.

-Flowform vessels provide not only a means of demonstrating the phenomenon of rhythmically pulsing water artistically, they also enable a wide range of applications influencing biological

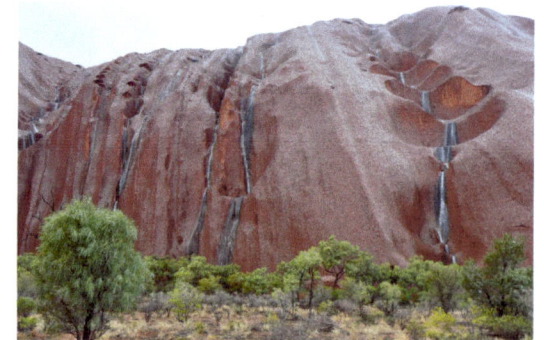

Rainfall at Uluru, erosion patterns reflecting the rhythmic pulsating movement of water, reproduced in the "Flowform" design

103

33 Flowform Water
Research 1970-2007 (J.
Schwuchow, J. Wilkes
et al) Healing Water
Foundation 2008

34 The True Power of
Water- Healing and
Discovering Ourselves
(Masaru Emoto) 2005
Beyond Words

and botanical processes through the rhythmical movement of water, remembering that all life processes are themselves always rhythmical. Thus artistic and technological applications can be combined in mutual harmony. [33]

"Flowform" cascades have been shown to improve the quality of water in many circumstances, after treatment through gravel filters and reed bed, the passage through the flow form will regenerate the water which can be returned to nature in a condition that is beneficial to the environment. There has been a noticeable improvement in the health of plants and animals in the vicinity of -Flowform- cascades.

The life-giving quality of water in its natural state has been described by Masaru Emoto in his book -The True Power of Water, Healing and Discovering Ourselves-. Using high-speed photography of water molecules at the moment they freeze. The energetic quality of the water is then assessed by analysing the ice crystals. We can see in a photo the crystallisation of water taken from a bottle on which was strapped a mobile phone in transmission-reception mode, the crystal thus generated is misshapen and of poor quality, while another taken from a bottle placed between speakers playing Bach's "Toccata and Fugue in D minor" shows a rich and complex six-sided crystal. [34]

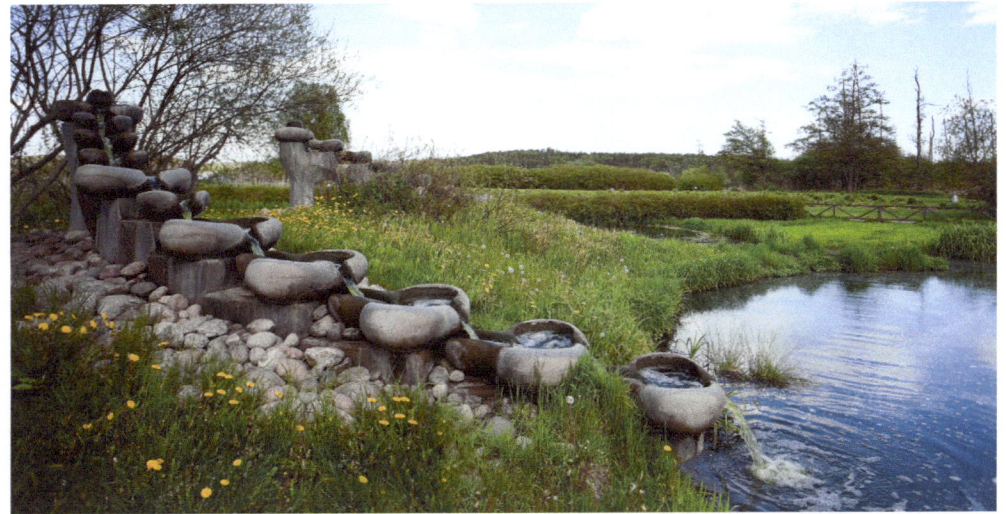

"Flowform" Cascades reproduce the natural pulsating rhythm of water in the landscape

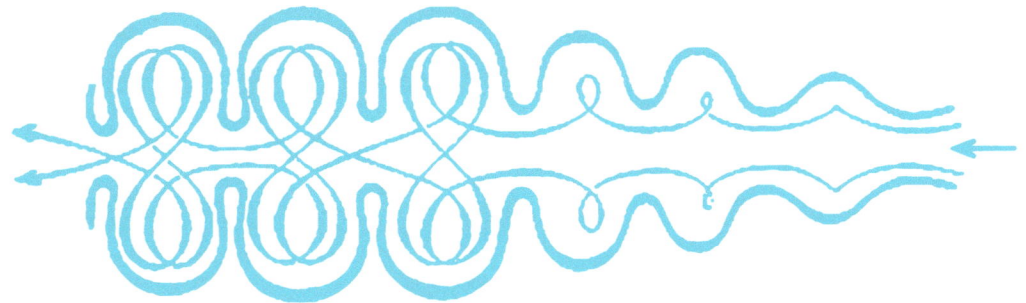

The pulsating patterns generated by the "Flowform" cascades, are similar to the natural movements of liquids inside living organisms

09 /
Landscaping

The ability to appreciate the landscape on all three levels enriches the soul.

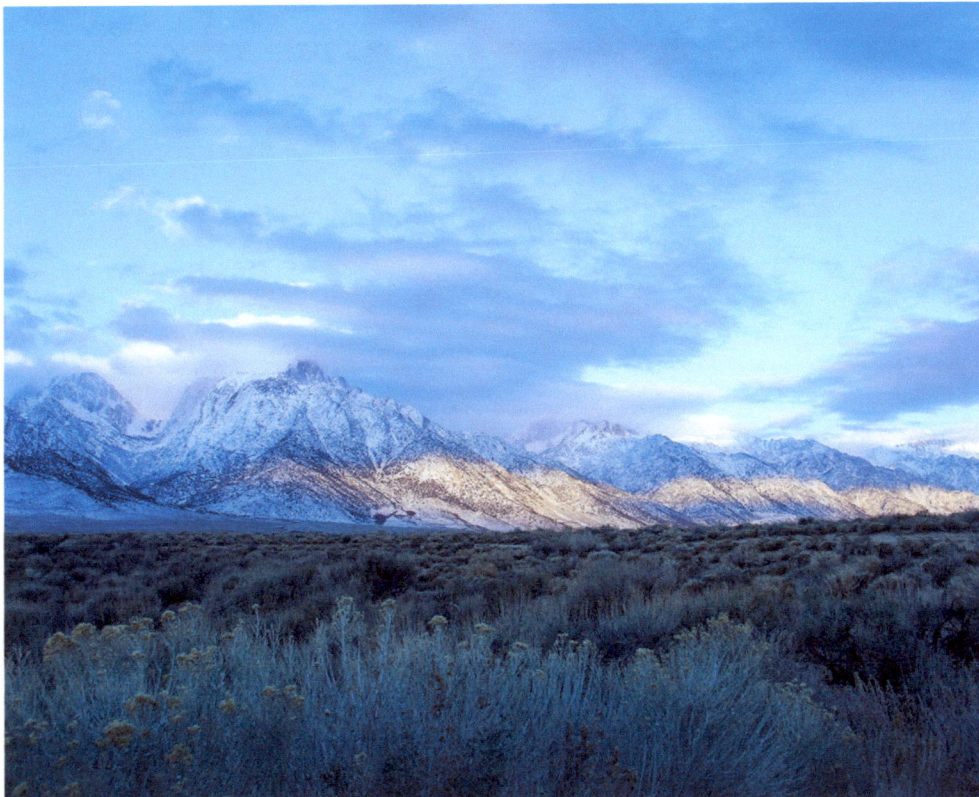

EMOTIONAL IMPACT

The emotional and aesthetic impact of a landscape is proportional to its diversity and is perceived on three distinct levels.

1. The macro scale: the pattern of hills, forests and scenery.

2. The meso scale: the specific areas of local vegetation.

3. The micro scale: the individual species of plants and trees within a given area.

In order to offer the inhabitants, the possibility of appreciating the landscape on all three levels, particular care will need to be taken when positioning the residential areas, the roads, the parks and other man-made infrastructure. The availability of the macro scale and the meso scale is often absent in most suburban developments, houses are fenced in and the close proximity of neighbours blocks the view, which often induces a feeling of claustrophobia.

There is also the economic factor, most well-situated sites, offering the best views, are very expensive. It is still possible to create spaces of beauty and tranquillity in small backyards or even courtyards. Many cultures offer examples of small sacred spaces such as the Zen garden in Japan or the Balinese garden with its family shrine.

106

THE GARDEN AS A HEALING AND SACRED SPACE

The private garden is one of the last bastions where almost unlimited creativity can be expressed in a suburban space, it is not subject to building by-laws and with a small budget and determination one can achieve a lot.

It is easier to proceed when there is a clear plan to follow, we can start with planning and designing on the Symbolic Level, the Energy Level and finally the Physical Level:

The Symbolic Level:

This will determine the nature and purpose of the garden, will it be a space for meditation and contemplation, an area for recreation and exercise, or a combination of the two.

Will it be connected to the landscape at large and to the cosmos or should it be self-contained and introvert?

First the space needs to be connected to its environment, the way we access it: is it open as if it was a natural extension of the living area, is it constricted with a narrow passage, a step or threshold to suggest a transition, a birth into a higher vibration, often a path and even a small labyrinth built with a different texture takes the visitor from the mundane to the sacred.

A path, a hedge or a statue can be oriented towards the rising sun at the solstice or equinox. The sunrise direction can also be personalised to resonate with the inhabitants, like their birthday, anniversary or saint day. The shapes of flower beds can be inspired by sacred geometry to enhance features such as fountains, ponds or lanterns. Shrines dedicated to deities or threshold to suggest a transition, a birth into a higher vibration, nature symbols can provide a focus to a sacred garden.

The Energy Level:

Once the basic layout is established we can flesh out the design using the interplay of the tellurian energies to bestow on the garden, the feeling we wish to resonate with:

Fire Energies

The fire energies are expressed by:
• Lantern, torches
• Red flowers

Water Energies

To honour water use:
• Ponds
• Fountains and bird baths

Air Energies

These are best enhanced with the following items:
• Rustling leaves plants such as bamboo
• Bells, chimes and flags

Earth Energies

The earth energies thrive in areas built with:
• Rockeries
• Pot plants

The Physical Level:

This will be likely determined by the lay of the land, the nature of the site, is it flat or sloping, rocky and dry or does it need to be drained, the use of local rocks and plants should be favoured to privilege the resonance of the garden with the local climate.

Garden design with Feng Shui principles:

Feng Shui offers a clear and simple set of guidelines to design and harmonise a garden, using the five elements.

Using the "controlling principle" and the "correcting principle" described in the "Five Elements" chapter, it is possible to balance all the elements in harmony with the climate, the geography, the seasons and even the inhabitants.

107

ELEMENTS	WOOD	FIRE	EARTH	METAL	WATER
DIRECTIONS	EAST	SOUTH	CENTRE	WEST	NORTH
FEATURES	WOOD ITEMS	BARBECUE	STATUES	PERGOLA	POND
	GREEN PLANTS	LIGHTS	ROCKERY	WIND CHIMES	FOUNTAIN
PLANTS	BAMBOO	RED FLOWERS	POT PLANTS	WHITE FLOWERS	GREENHOUSE
SHAPES	VERTICAI	POINTED	HORIZONTAL	CIRCLE	WAVY

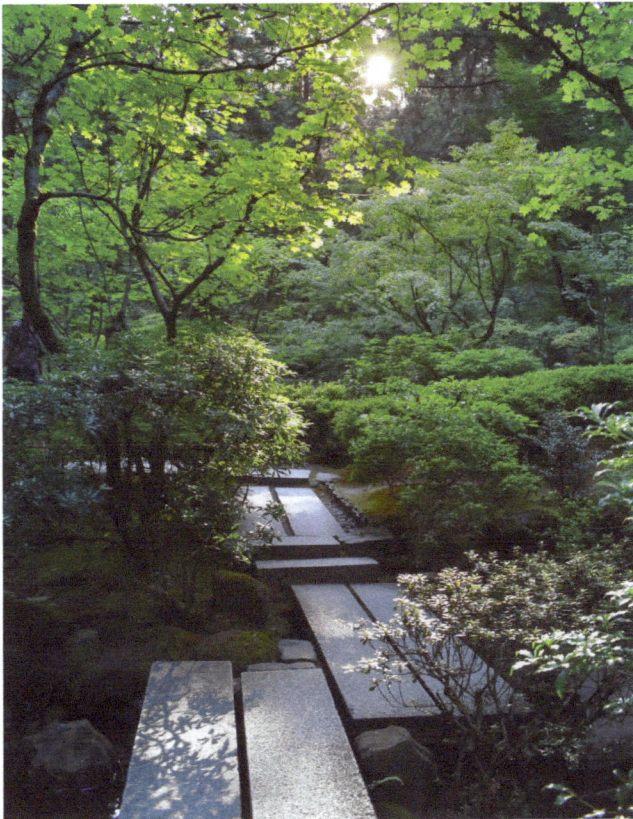

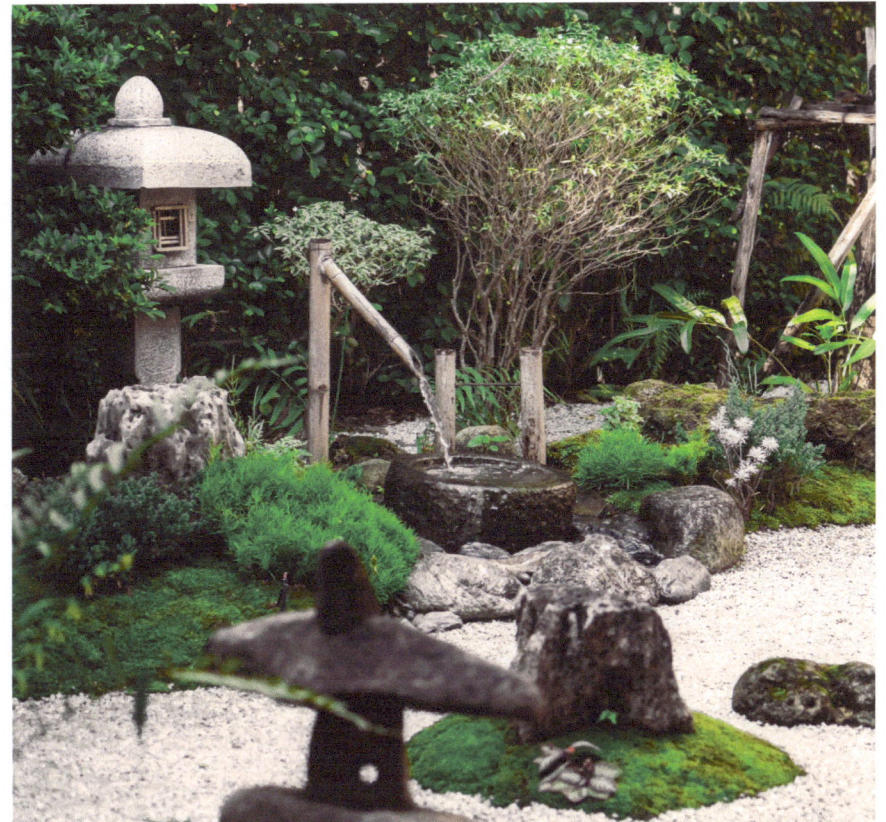

108

BIODIVERSITY

Landscaping design is a prime consideration and one of the most important influences in the health of the environment. It plays a vital role in generating biodiversity, augmenting the richness and variety of species and their interaction with the environment.

Biodiversity characterises the relationship of many different habitats each with its particular flora and fauna. These parts form a complex ecosystem. Its complexity is its strength and guaranties its stability, resilience and its resistance against adverse conditions.

Furthermore, biodiversity promotes richness of species and genetic variability; it is closely linked and dependent on landscape design.

Landscaping should provide a bridge between the requirement to support a diversity of species and the emotional perception of the environment.

The use of local plants is a great step to promote and sustain biodiversity, even in a very small garden, insects and birds will thrive and enhance the quality of the space.

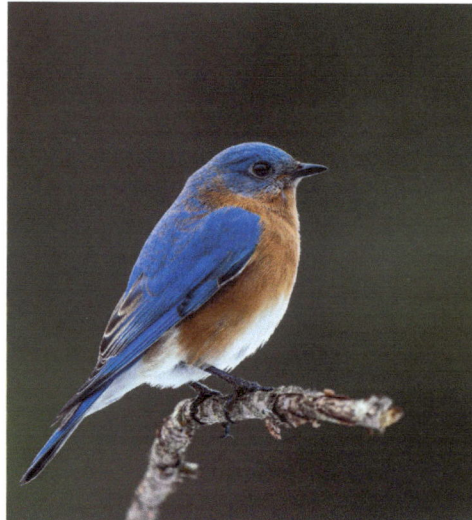

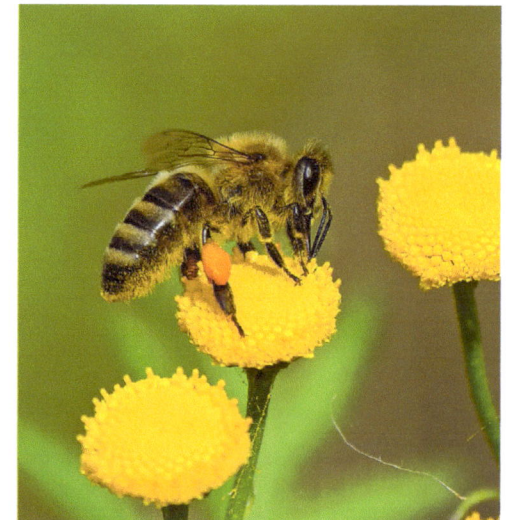

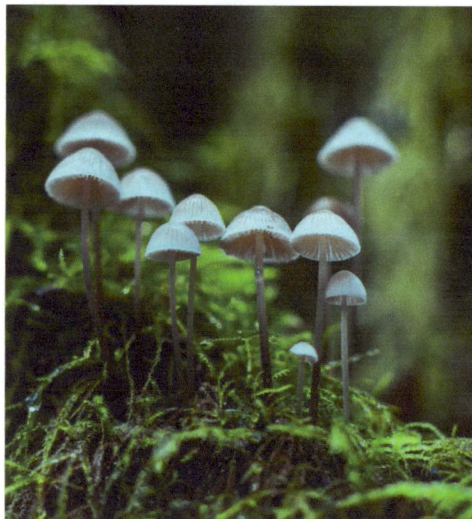

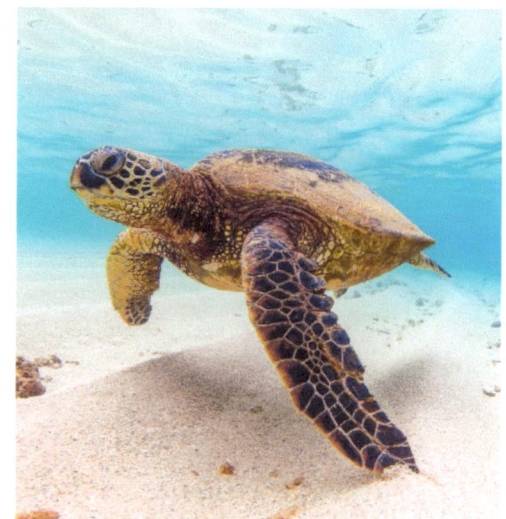

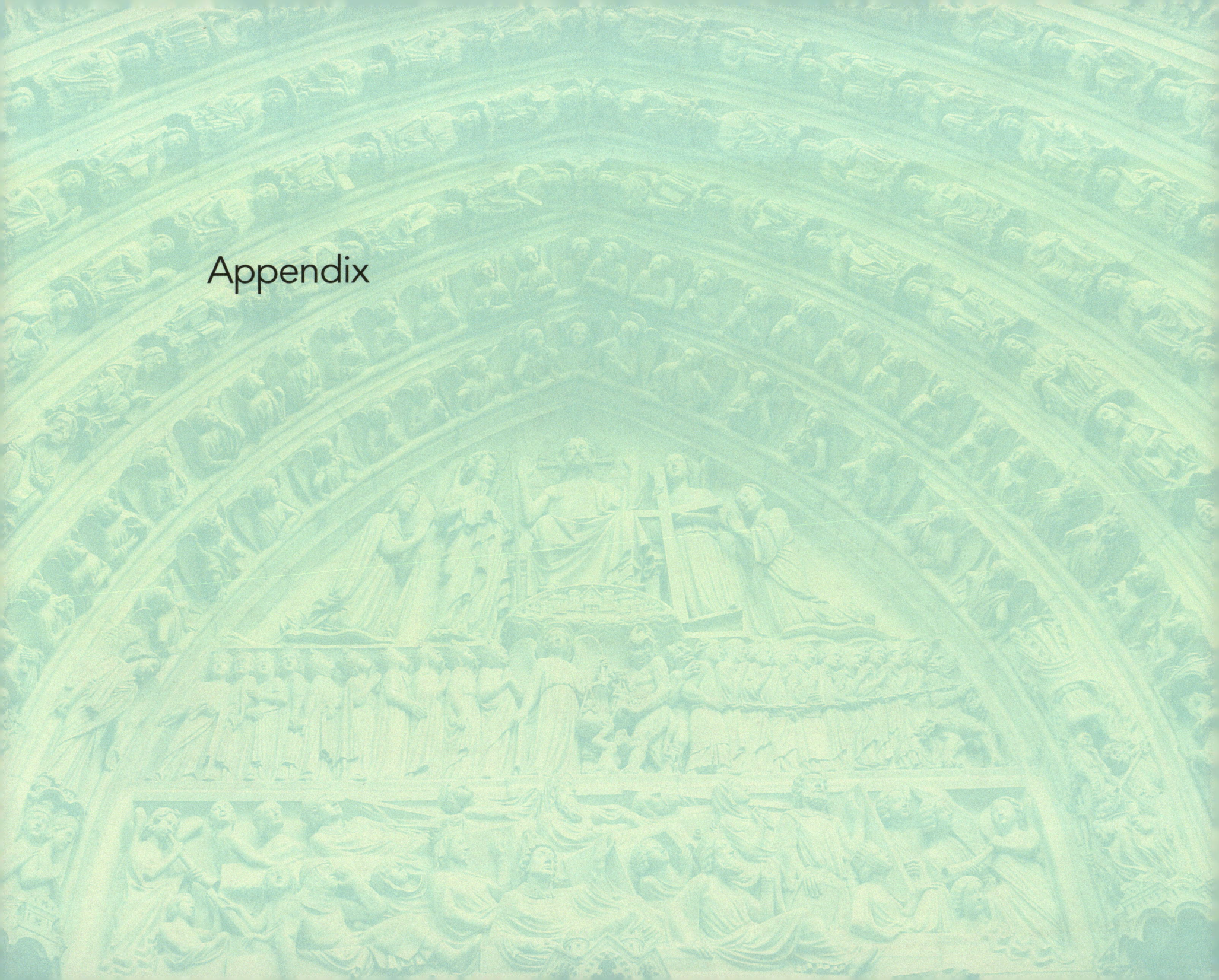

Appendix

MAGIC SQUARES

A square is said to be magic when the numbers that are composing it add up to the same total horizontally, vertically and diagonally.

They have been used in almost every culture. In China, the magic squares were called "Lo Shu" and the square of three pattern was said to have been found on the back of a turtle by the emperor Yu.

The magic squares represent in their numerology the characteristics of the seven astrological planets, the Sun, the Moon, Mars, Mercury, Jupiter, Venus and Saturn.

It is only around the year 1000 that Arab numbers started to be used in Western Europe; previously letters had a numeric value. Originally the squares were composed of letters be it Sanskrit, Hebrew, Greek or Roman. The Greek square was composed of seven vowels; each vowel was related to a planet and a musical note. They were used as protecting talismans.

The act of organising numbers in a particular order was seen as an act of magic resulting in a particular vibration resonating with various aspects of the universe, planets, metals, gemstones and days of the week. Their ability to resonate with these different aspects was used to harmonise the energies of certain areas or certain buildings. It was a way to bring into the construction process the essence of these higher principles and their attributes.

Each one of the seven wonders of the world was said to resonate with a Magic square, The Pharos, or lighthouse of Alexandria with the square of Saturn, the Temple of Zeus at Olympia with the square of Jupiter, the Hanging gardens of Babylon with the square of Mars, the Colossus of Rhodes with the square of the Sun, the Mausoleum of Halicarnassus with the square of Venus, the pyramids of Egypt with the square of Mercury and the temple of Diana at Ephesus with the square of the Moon.

♄ **SEAL OF SATURN (LEAD)**

Square of 3 Total 15

4	9	2
3	5	7
8	1	6

♃ **SEAL OF JUPITER (TIN)**

Square of 4 Total 34

4	14	15	1
9	7	6	12
5	11	10	8
16	2	3	13

♂ **SEAL OF MARS (IRON)**

Square of 5 Total 65

11	24	7	20	3
4	12	25	8	16
17	5	13	21	9
10	18	1	14	22
23	6	19	2	15

Apart from their symbolic significance, the magic squares were also used to define and calculate harmonious proportions for many ancient buildings.

If we were to link all the multiple of 3 on the Seal of Mars we would obtain the pattern shown below:

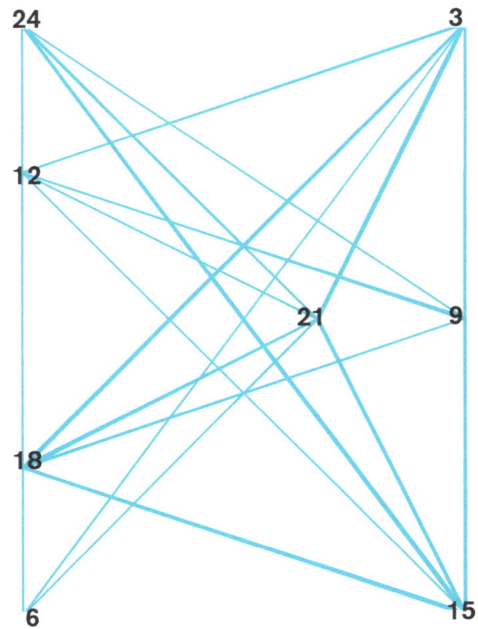

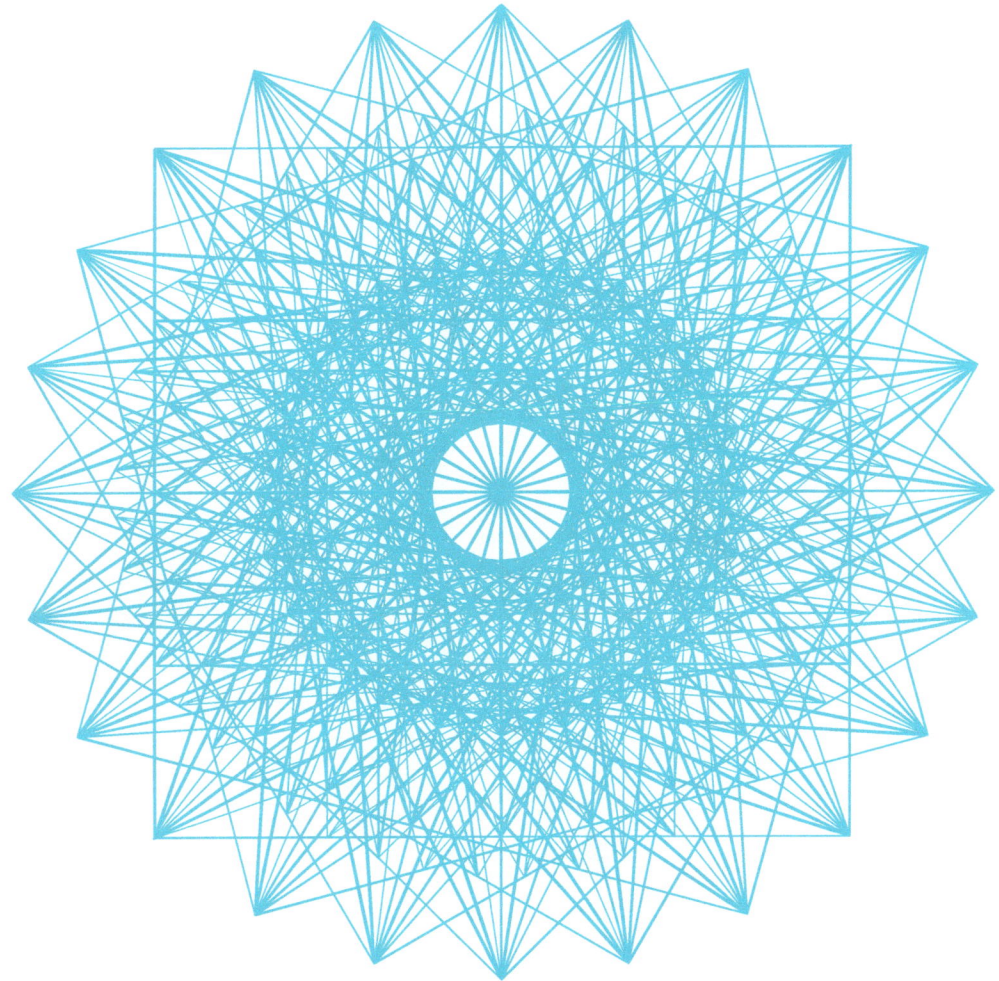

Above is shown the pattern generated by linking all the multiples of 3 on the Seal of Mars. This pattern is then rotated every 15 degrees.

⊙ **SEAL OF THE SUN**
(GOLD)

Square of 6 Total 111

6	32	3	34	35	1
7	11	27	28	8	30
19	14	16	15	23	24
18	20	22	21	17	13
25	29	10	9	26	12
36	5	33	4	2	31

☿ **SEAL OF MERCURY**
(MERCURY)

Square of 7 Total 175

22	47	16	41	10	35	4
5	23	48	17	42	11	29
30	6	24	49	18	36	12
13	31	7	25	43	19	37
38	14	32	1	26	44	20
21	39	8	33	2	27	45
46	15	40	9	34	3	28

♀ **SEAL OF VENUS**
(COPPER)

Square of 8 Total 260

8	58	59	5	4	62	63	1
49	15	14	52	53	11	10	56
41	23	22	44	45	19	18	48
23	34	35	29	28	38	39	25
40	26	27	37	36	30	31	33
17	47	46	20	21	43	42	24
9	55	54	12	13	51	50	16
64	2	3	61	60	6	7	57

☾ **SEAL OF THE MOON**
(SILVER)

Square of 9 Total 369

37	78	29	70	21	62	13	54	5
6	38	79	30	71	22	63	14	46
47	7	39	80	31	72	23	55	15
16	48	8	40	81	32	64	24	56
57	17	49	9	41	73	33	65	25
26	58	18	50	1	42	74	34	66
67	27	59	10	51	2	43	75	35
36	68	19	60	11	52	3	44	76
77	28	69	20	61	12	53	4	45

	1	1	1	1	1	1	1	1	1		
1	1	2	3	4	5	6	7	8	9	45	=9
1	2	4	6	8	1	3	5	7	9	45	=9
1	3	6	9	3	6	9	3	6	9	45	=9
1	4	8	3	7	2	6	1	5	9	45	=9
1	5	1	6	2	7	3	8	4	9	45	=9
1	6	3	9	6	3	9	6	3	9	45	=9
1	7	5	3	1	8	6	4	2	9	45	=9
1	8	7	6	5	4	3	2	1	9	45	=9
1	9	9	9	9	9	9	9	9	9	45	=9
	45	45	54	45	45	54	45	45	81	459	=18
	=9	=9	=9	=9	=9	=9	=9	=9	=9		=9

THE VEDIC SQUARE

It is basically a 9-multiplication table where the result is placed in the corresponding cell. When the result is more than 2 digits, it is reduced to 1, for example, 5 x 5 equals 25, thus 2+5 equal 7.

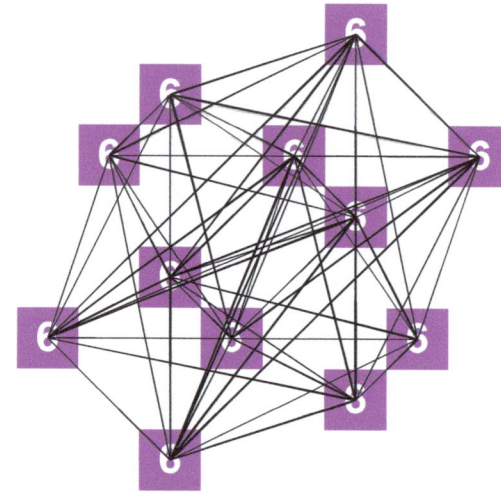

The Vedic Square has been used to generate Islamic design patterns often seen in mosques and palaces such as the octagonal dome of the Alhambra in Cordoba, Spain. In the Vedic square shown above it is fascinating to observe the distribution of the numbers across the board. Every line or column adds up to 45, 54 or 81 which can all be reduced to 9 and the grand total is 459 which, when reduced becomes 18 then 9. Furthermore, if we observe the pattern generated by the distribution of the number 1, we can see that it is the mirror of the pattern generated by the number 8, the total of these mirrored patterns is 9, the pattern generated by 2s is mirrored by the 7s

115

for a total of 9. It is the same for the 4s and 5s and the 3s and 6s which also add up to 9.

We can see the pattern generated by connecting all the 6s in the Vedic Square. We can then rotate this pattern around its axis and superimpose them all to build up a blueprint for a mosaic or a carved ceiling.

This process is described by David Saltman (Decoding Arabic Design) in "Shelter":

1 Decoding Arabic Design (David Saltman) Shelter 1973 (Shelter publications)

The method of simplification is really elegant in my opinion. When you actually do this business of laying the nets over one another, you find that many of the lines just coalesce in a black blob. The blobs stay in the final design. You also get the effect where a 20-sided figure approaches a circle, which may be rendered into a circle in the end or may just stay a 20-sided figure. Sometimes everything within one of these circles is erased, and the line segments left over are connected with one another with yet another numerical code.[1]

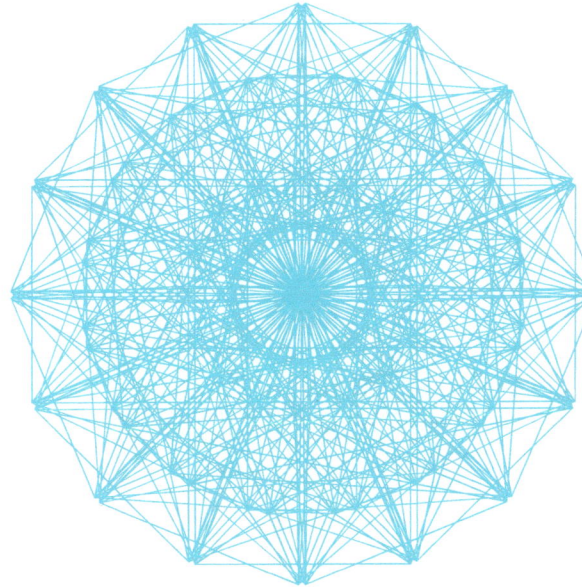

"Blueprint" generated by rotating the "6" net 22.5 degrees around its centre.

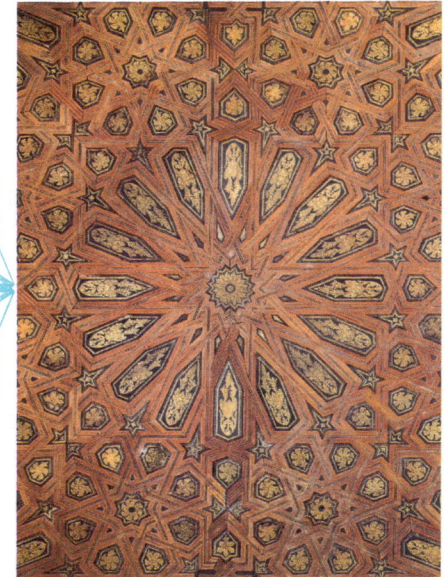

Carved wooden ceiling in the Alhambra

FORM-FIELDS (Shape caused waves)

We usually see form as having an aesthetic or a functional quality. Unless we are gifted with a certain sensitivity, we do not conceive that shapes, in their very essence have a power which is radiating in the environment. The architect- priests of ancient civilisations used different shapes and architectural forms to either elevate the souls of the worshipers in temples or to protect tombs and sacred sites. The French poet Charles Baudelaire gives us an intuitive insight into the magic world of shapes when he writes, "Every shape created by man is eternal, because form is independent of matter and is not constituted of molecules."

The radiation generated by forms, or Form Field, could be seen as the aura generated by various shapes which affects us on a subtle level. In its grossest form, it could manifest itself as our aesthetic judgement of a particular shape. In its more subtle aspect, it would speak to our very soul and, depending on the quality or purpose of the object, we could be affected positively or negatively.

The expression "Form Field" is translated from the French term -Ondes de formes- used by the researchers Leon Chaumery and Andre de Belizal.[2]

De Belizal explains that Form Fields are generated by geometrical shapes which capture cosmo- tellurian radiation and, as these forms become saturated, they radiate in the environment.

In his work with his colleague P. A. Morel, de Belizal[3] writes "Beside the field of natural radiation, there exist other vibrations generated by the very shape of matter. Effectively absolutely everything in the universe radiates and emits vibrations. Some of these vibrations have a level of oscillation so minute as to escape the detection of our best instruments. The microscopic frequency of these vibrations is their very strength".

"These Form Fields are situated in the spectrum which encompasses all the radiation existing in the cosmos".

It is assumed the vibratory rate or the wavelength of Form Fields is shorter than light. As Jean de la Foye[4], a colleague of de Belizal writes -Form Fields have an influence on our health. They vibrate in resonance with living cells which act as small resonators-.

Every structure or shape modifies the totality of the cosmo- tellurian field through its form nature and volume.

In a book about "The power of shapes surrounding us" Bernard Baudouin[5] lists the nature and properties of Form fields:

- Form Fields are generated by every existing shape and penetrate each other.

- Unlike other known radiation Form Fields keep the same intensity whatever the distance between the point of emission and the site of reception.

- All architectural monuments, built of natural material such as stone, can be powerful emitters of Form Fields.

- Form Fields can be concentrated or focused with a convex wooden lens.

- Most materials have the ability to be charged with the radiation of Form Fields. Apparently heat (over 64 degrees Celsius) can destroy the charge.

- The capacity of penetration of Form Fields can be very high. No material, whatever its thickness, seems to be able to stop them. They can however be stopped by other shapes such as woven textile or metallic webs.

- It is possible to generate Form Fields artificially by creating different shapes and to control the intensity and direction of emission.

2 L. Chaumery & A. de Belizal (Essai de radiesthésie vibratoire) Desforges

3 A. de Belizal & P. A. Morel (Physique microvibratoire et forces invisibles) Desforges

4 J. de la Foye (Ondes de vie ondes de mort) Laffont

5 B. Baudouin (Le pouvoir des formes qui nous entourent) Tchou

Form field emission related to different beam shapes

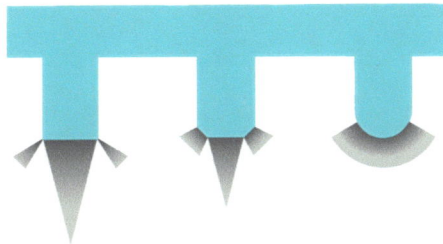

Right angle   Chamfered   Rounded

Form field emission related to different wall angles

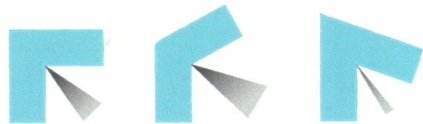

Right angle   Obtuse angle   Acute abgle

The repetition of a particular shape will amplify its effect

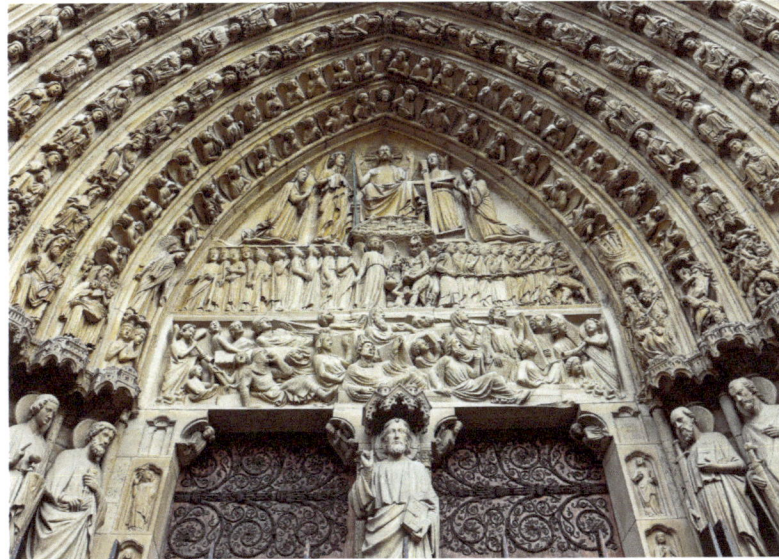

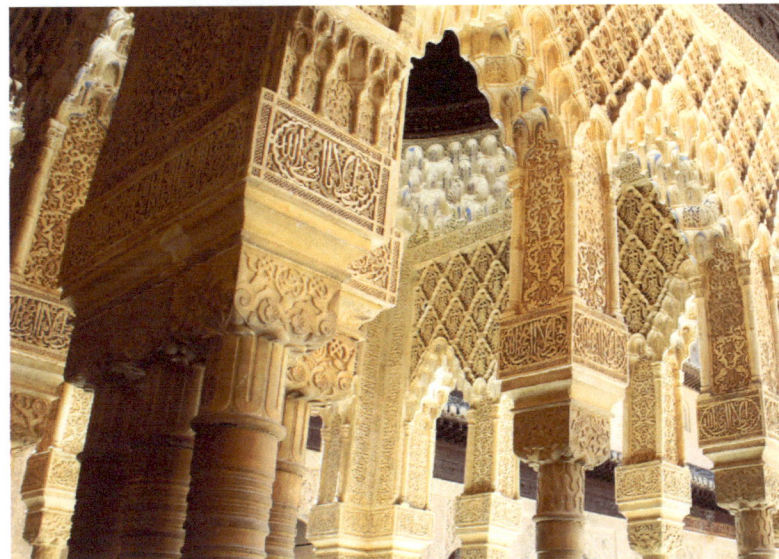

Visible colour spectrum

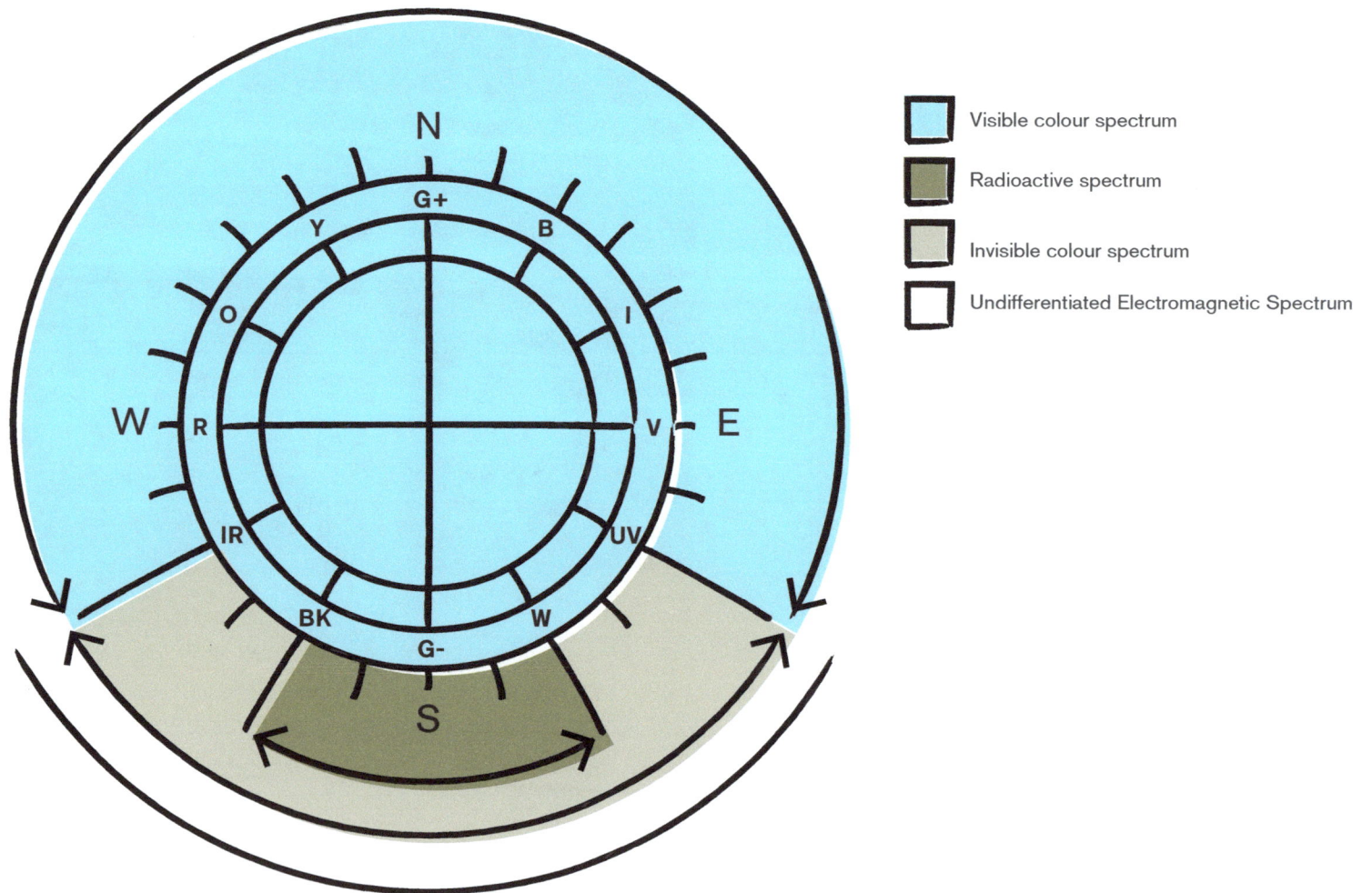

Visible colour spectrum

Radioactive spectrum

Invisible colour spectrum

Undifferentiated Electromagnetic Spectrum

119

GOLDEN MEAN DETAILED CALCULATIONS

In the Golden Section the smaller segment (d) is to the bigger segment (D) as the latter is to the total of both.

So, d: D = D: (D + d) this ratio corresponds to the ratio of the side of the decagon to its radius. The decagon generates geometrical progressions of the Golden section.

The pentagram, a magical symbol, also gener-ates the Golden Section dimensions.

The dimensions of the Pythagorean triangles drawn in a rectangle within a circle offer a progression of harmonious ratios near to the Golden Section. 1-2-3-5-8 (Fibonacci series).

When Phi (Φ), the Golden Section is squared it becomes the same number increased by one unit (1.618 square = 2.618), and when divided into unit it is the same number minus one (1: 1.618 = 0.618).

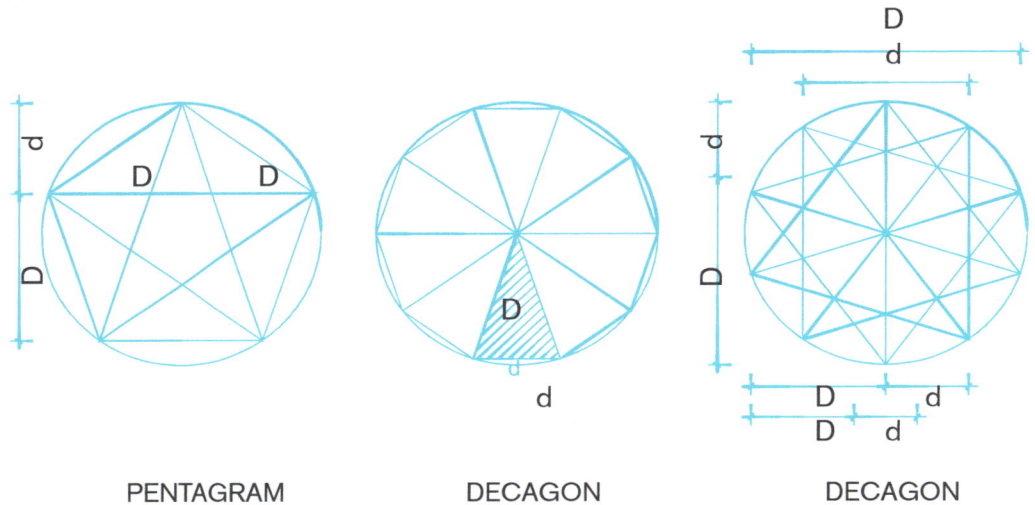

PENTAGRAM

DECAGON

DECAGON

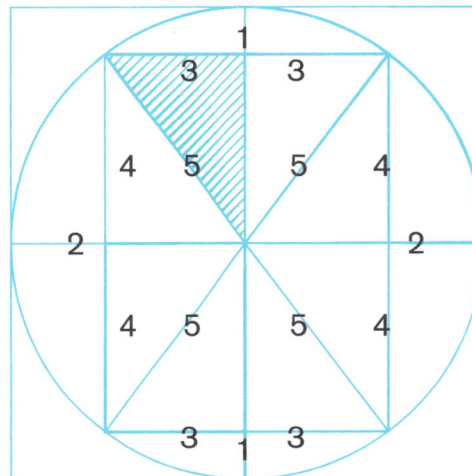

Pythagorean triangles within a circle

Geometry and the Golden Section

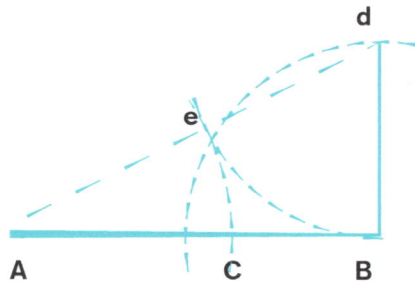

Knowing **AC** find **B**:

From **C** draw the perpendicular **f** such as **Cf = AC**. From **g** in the middle of **AC** draw a circle with the radius **Gf** cutting **AC** in **B**.

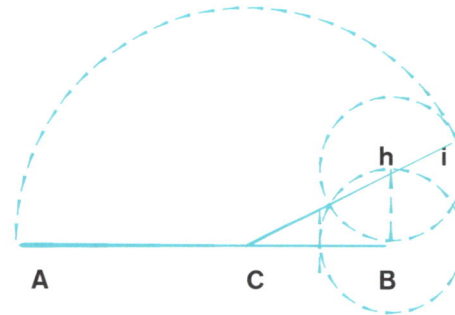

Knowing **AB** find **C**:

Bd is perpendicular to **AB** such as **dB = AB/2**

Connect **Ad** and report, from **d**, **dB** on **Ad** to determine **e**. Report **Ae**, from **A**, on **AB** to find **C**.

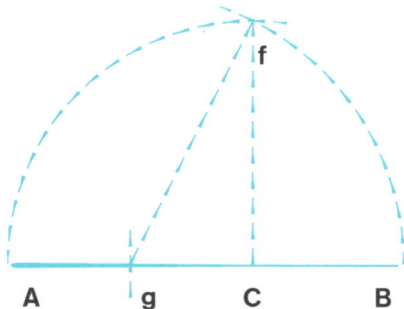

Knowing **CB** find **A**:

Draw **hB** as a perpendicular to **CB** such as **hB= CB/2**.

Using **h** as a centre draw a circle with the radius **hB** cutting **Ch** in **i**. **C** is the centre of a circle with the radius **Ci** cutting **CB** in **A**.

121

Before the phenomena of Nature, it is necessary to observe, to study and to be astonished by nothing.

– Gottfried W. Leibnitz

RADIESTHESIA, THE ART OF DOWSING

DOWSING ON THE MOUNTAINS

As a young architect working in a ski resort in Switzerland I participated in the design and the construction of a restaurant at the end station of a ski lift on top of a mountain.

We advised the client, it happened to be the local city council, that we needed a geological survey of the site to see if water could be found nearby for the restaurant. We were promptly answered that it would be too expensive and unnecessary. They would ask the local dowser to come on the site. I was surprised, after the dowser had given his results, the exact spot where to dig, the depth and even the predicted flow, to see that he was so trusted that our client immediately ordered a helicopter with the drilling equipment to be flown on site the next days. The water flowed as indicated.

PRINCIPLES

Radiesthesia is still the best-known way to determine the position of geomagnetic grids such as the Hartmann grid and the Peyre grid as well as a very reliable tool to find water and geological faults.

According to the Abbot Alexis Mermet (1866-1937) priest of Jussy (Switzerland) near Geneva, who was recognised as one of the best dowsers of the last century, three persons out of four can dowse. It is an innate ability that every human possesses and it can be success-fully taught even to those who do not show a natural predisposition to it.

The basic principles of radiesthesia as explained by Alexis Mermet are the following:

i) All bodies without exception are constantly emitting undulations or radiations.

ii) The human body enters these fields of influence and becomes the seat of nervous reactions, of some kind of current which flows through the hand.

iii) If an appropriate object such as a rod or a pendulum is held in the hand, the invisible flux is made manifest in the movement given to this object which acts as a kind of indicator.

He often uses the phenomenon of resonance to further explain the effect of dowsing.

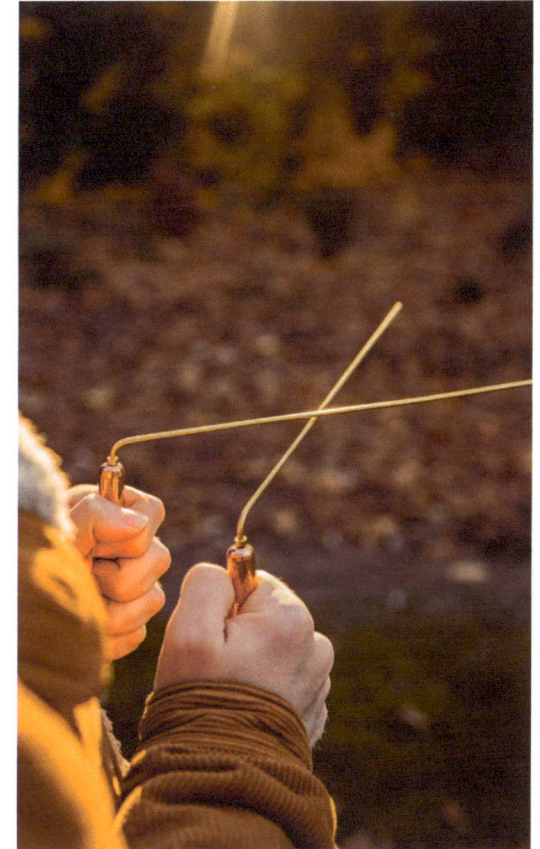

122

6 Principles and
Practice of Radiesthesia
(Abbe Mermet) Element
Books 1987

7 A.M. Bell -Practical
Dowsing, A Symposium-
(G. Bell & Sons London
1965)

*"When a dowser stands on a site containing any mineral ore, such as gold for example (Atomic number 79), the radiation of this gold causes traces of gold naturally present in the radiesthetist organism to vibrate in resonance and emits cellular radiations which, manifesting as a function of the atomic number of gold, are detected by the organism and move the pendulum. The same applies to all the substances contained in the soil for our organism contains all the simple bodies of chemistry."*6

HOW TO DEVELOP OUR MAGNETISM:

*The beginner can rely on the experience of others only to a very limited extent as there are no universally known methods of dowsing. Each practitioner will develop his own technique from experience, as well as the choice of their own tools.*7

When looking for water, the Hartmann grid or to determine the quality of tellurian energies, we use our body as an antenna and an amplifier of signals. Our ability to dowse is then determined by the quality of the receptors situated in our body. According to Yves Roccard these receptors are composed of minuscule particles of magnetite and are found in different areas of the body, two behind the superciliary arches, two in the neck, one in each elbow, two in the lower back, one behind each knee and one under each foot. Several factors will influence the quality of these magnetite receptors.

Many different theories have been put forward to explain dowsing, whether it is resonance (Alexis Mermet), tiny magnetite receptors (Yves Roccard) or, as some others think the adrenal or pineal glands, dowsing still remains very much a mystery. The only certainty is that results are consistently and successfully obtained.

Balanced diet

The ideal diet would be rich in energy and composed of fruit and vegetables organically grown and eaten raw or juiced. Food which has been overcooked, microwaved, tinned or chemically treated is dead and is not a good energy source, it can even be energy depleting and weaken the body's resistance to diseases.

Rest

It is important to be well rested and free of stress. The bed should be in a healthy spot free of electromagnetic pollution with the head oriented north. Choose preferably a bed and natural fibre bedding.

Clothing

It is preferable to wear clothes that are not too tight and made of natural fibres. The colours should be suited to your personality and stimulate your energy. Synthetic clothing accumulates static electricity and causes disturbances and losses in your energy field. When dowsing it is recommended to take off all jewellery, watches.

Massages

Our energy body just like its physical counterpart, needs to be alive and vibrant. It can be stimulated and revitalised with self-massage. First one can massage the areas where the receptors are found.

Shiatsu applied to oneself is called Do In, the purpose of this Japanese massage technique is to stimulate the path of energy throughout our body. These paths are called meridians.

Focussing exercises

Before dowsing, especially when beginning, it is helpful to put oneself in a different frame of mind than the usual day to day life. It is like fine tuning our "body's antennae" and opening them to a finer and more subtle type of sensory stimulus.

Standing in a quiet place, facing north, feet apart, breathe deeply. Rub the hands together until warm, and then, with palms facing each other, feel the warmth and energy generated by the hands as they are spread further and further apart. Then slowly draw them together again.

Avoiding energy losses

Emotional stress, negative thinking, substance abuse, polluted environment, are all causes of energy loss.

Recharging exercises

After dowsing on site, looking for water or the Hartmann grid, the body can feel tired and depleted of energy. Sunbathing is an effective way of renewing one's energy, so is walking bare foot in the early morning dew, or gentle breathing exercises in nature facing north, aligned with the geomagnetic field.

DOWSING TOOLS:

Ultimately the experienced and sensitive dowser does not need any kind of rod or pendulum, the hand can detect by itself any disturbance of the magnetic field, these hands can even heal others. It is therefore not necessary to acquire expensive and complicated detection equipment. It is more advantageous to make instruments adapted to one's needs and to develop one's own sensitivity.

Divining rod or dowsing rod

The divining rod is one of the oldest ways known to man to find underground water. It is a forked stick which can be made of wood (hazel or willow) or metal and used to locate water, minerals or other material underground. The rod is grasped lightly by its two forks and held with the end facing forward. The divining rod moves downward or upward independently when one walks directly over water or other substances.

Pendulum

Dowsing with a pendulum was practised in ancient Egypt, some stoneware pendulums have been found in tombs in the Valley of the Kings.

According to experienced dowsers, the material chosen to make a pendulum is a matter of personal choice and preference. They can be made of wood, glass, crystal, amber, stone or different metal. Lead, however, is known to absorb certain radiation which could be detrimental where research needs to be conducted with a tool as neutral as possible. It needs to be regularly washed in clear water; another solution is to paint the lead white.

8 Enel -La Trilogie de la Rota- (Dervy Livres 1973)

The shape of the pendulum will have some influence in dowsing. It is preferable to have regular shapes, the sphere is a good universal pendulum, a pointed pendulum will favour work on plans. Some researchers have developed a variety of pendulums for specific tasks, such as the "fictitious cone" pendulum used to detect the quality of form fields. Invented by Andre de Belizal and Leon Chaumery, a disk slides along an axis forming a more or less elongated abstract cone between the tip of the pendulum and the edge of the disk. The axis is graduated in 12 equal intervals assigned to each colour of the *"undifferentiated electromagnetic spectrum"* as defined by Enel.8 This spectrum is also called *"negative green spectrum"* by A. de Belizal and P. A. Morel.

The weight of the pendulum is a matter of personal preference. Working with a light pendulum does not require as much energy as a heavier one and is more sensitive. However too much sensitivity might be difficult to handle, especially for beginners. A heavier pendulum will avoid secondary reactions or unwanted interferences.

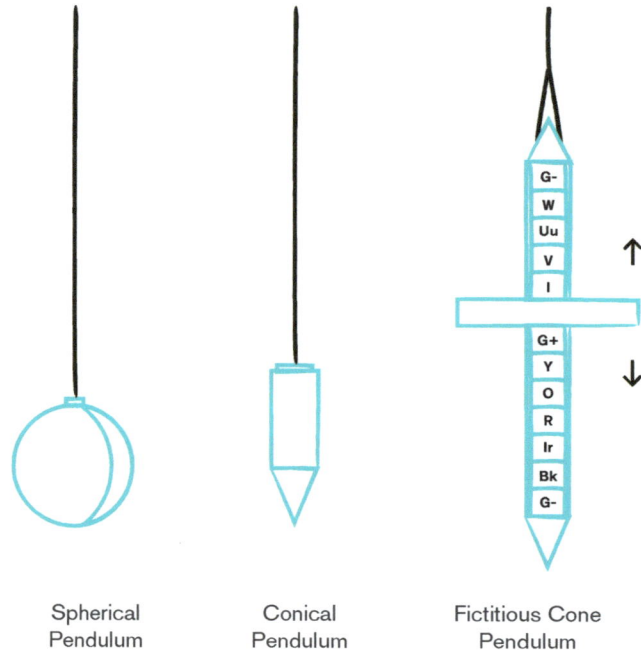

Spherical
Pendulum

Conical
Pendulum

Fictitious Cone
Pendulum

300

150

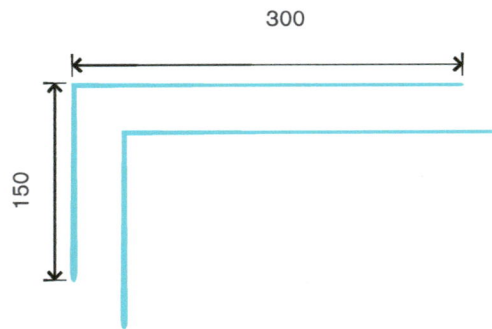

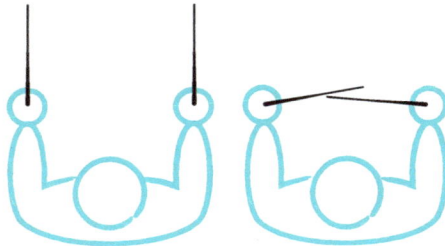

The pendulum should be held without stress and effort. A good support would be a small chain or a cotton string which slides easily between the fingers to vary the length.

Parallel rods or L rods

Parallel rods or "German rods" are widely used by geobiologists to locate the Hartmann grid.

They are usually made of brass (Ø5mm) 450 mm long and bent at a right angle 150mm from the end.

They are easy to use by beginners. They can be also used for dowsing.

When working on a large site to locate ley lines or water veins, heavier, bigger (Ø5-6mm) and less sensitive rods should be used, the total length being up to 900mm, with the angle situated at 300mm.

To make the operation easier, the way the parallel rods are held can vary according to the type of research and take into account the work on three distinct levels, as defined in geobiology -physical level, energy level and symbolic or spiritual level-. When working on the physical level, the rods should be held slightly under the navel. When working on the energy level the rods should be at the solar plexus height, and at the height of the heart when doing a search related to the symbolic or spiritual level.

The rods are held loosely, parallel to each other. The dowser walks slowly over the site or in a house and, the rods move towards each other when passing over a "wall" of the Hartmann grid or whatever other anomaly one is looking for.

9 Babonneau- Laflèche-
Martin (Traite de
Géobiologie) Edition
de l'Aire Lausanne

STARTING UP DOWSING:

Basic pendulum movements

Dowsing is usually practised with the active hand, which means the right hand for the right-handed and the left for the left-handed.

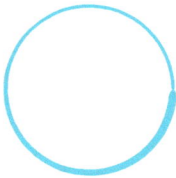

The first step is to determine one's natural pendulum movement, whether clockwise or anticlockwise. To do so, place the swinging pendulum over a perfectly drawn circle, soon the pendulum will start to rotate either clockwise or anticlockwise. This determines our positive polarity so a rotation in the opposite direction will indicate a negative polarity or answer.

It is easier to start dowsing with a moving pendulum -it saves energy and it is simple to observe the different changes in the movement of the

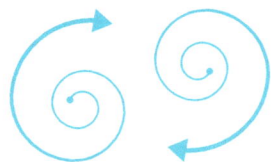

Try swinging your pendulum about 1cm over the figures above. It should rotate effortlessly in the same direction as the arrow. Go from one figure to the other and notice how the pendulum changes direction.

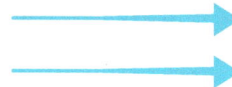

The figure above will induce a strong lateral swinging movement when the pendulum is placed immediately above, notice the changes as you move from one figure to the next.

Sometimes the pendulum stays absolutely immobile. This can be observed when placing the pendulum above the centre of a cross.

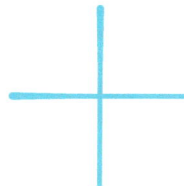

When the pendulum is attracted to a point and inert, it could mean that it is detecting absolute neutrality, such as a cross for example. It could also be a momentary interference or a lack of energy in the dowser.

Bibliography/
Photo credits

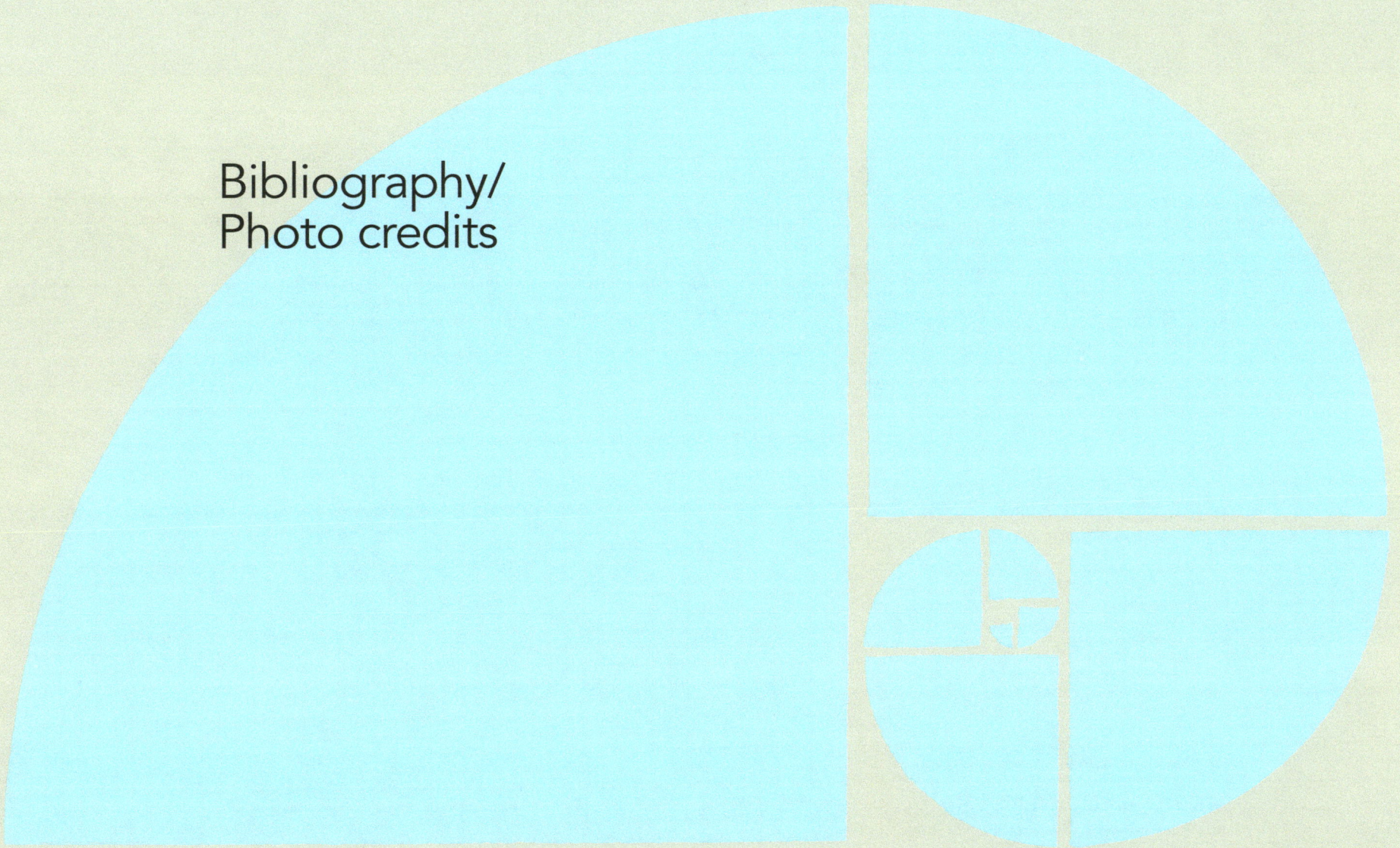

BIBLIOGRAPHY

James Lovelock (Gaia, The Practical Science of Planetary Medicine) 1991

Georges Lakhovsky (The Secret of Life) Tri State Press 1939 Jean-Paul Dillensenger (Habitation et sante- Eléments d'Architecture Biologique) Editions Dangles 1990

G. Altenbach-B. Legrais (Habitat et Sante) Ed. Cosmitel 1988

G. Altenbach-B. Legrais (Santé et Cosmo-tellurism) Ed. Dangles 1986

Nigel Pennick (The Ancient Science of Geomancy) CRCS Publications 1979

Frances A. Yates (The Art of Memory) The University of Chicago Press 1966

Jean de la Foye (Ondes de vie ondes de mort) Laffont 1975 Jean-Charles Fabre (Maisons entre Terre et Ciel) Arista Paris 1987

Eilert Ekwall (The Concise Oxford Dictionary of English Place Names) Clarendon Press

James R. Tyrrell (Australian Aboriginal Place Names and their meaning) Simmons Ltd. Glebe Sydney 1933

Elie Wiesel (Souls on Fire, Portraits and Legends of Hasidic Masters) Touchstone 1972

Decoding Arabic Design (David Saltman) Shelter 1973 D.Robins (The secret language of stone) Rider London 1988

B. Baudouin (Le pouvoir des formes qui nous entourent) Tchou- Editions Sand 1988

Rudolf Steiner (Anthroposophy and Science) Mercury Press 1991

Rudolf Steiner (Vers un Nouveau Style en Architecture) Triades

Rudolf Steiner (Nature des Couleurs) Editions Anthroposophiques Romandes 2009

Dr. Hans Jenny (Cymatics- A Study of Wave Phenomena & Vibration) Macromedia Press 2001

Rupert Sheldrake (A New Science of Life - The Hypothesis of Formative Causation) 1981

Anil Ananthaswamy (Ancient sound waves sculpted galaxy formation) The New Scientist 30th March 2012

Johannes Itten (The Elements of Color - A treatise on the colour system of Johannes Itten based on his book THE ART OF COLOUR) Van Nostrand Reinhold Company 1970

Wassily Kandinsky (On the spiritual in art) Salomon R. Guggenheim Foundation 1946

L. Chaumery & A. de Belizal (Essai de radiesthésie vibratoire) Desforges 1976

A. de Belizal & P. A. Morel (Physique micro-vibra-toire et forces invisibles) Desforges 1979

Y. Rocard (Le signal du sourcier) Dunod 1962

A. Lambert- P. Creuze (Etudes sur les influences cosmiques) Maison de la radiesthésie 1947

Dr. Quinquandon (12 Balles pour un Veto) Agriculture et vie 1974

A.M. Philips (Living with Electricity) - EM Fields Information Booklet No 1

Robert Endros (Le rayonnement de la terre et son influence sur la vie) Signal 1996

Grzegorz Redlarski et al. (The Influence of Electromagnetic Pollution on Living Organisms: Historical Trends and Forecasting Changes) BioMed Research International Volume 2015 Article 234098

Blanche Mertz (L'âme du lieu) Georg Geneva 1990

Vitruvius Pollio (The ten Books on Architecture) Harvard University Press 1914

Babonneau- Laflèche- Martin (Traité de Géobiologie) Editions de L'Aire Lausanne 1987

Stephen Skinner (The Living Earth Manual of Feng Shui) RKP London 1989

David Pearson (The Natural House Book) Collins Australia 1989

C. Braibant (Archipuncture) Maisons Saines Belgique 1988

Chuck Pettis (Secrets of Sacred Spaces- Discover and Create Places of Power) Llewellyn Publications 1999

Mark Balfour (The sign of the serpent, key to creative physics) Prism press 1990

Christopher Day (Places of the Soul - Architecture and Environmental Design as a Healing Art) Thorsons 1990

129

Robert Lawlor (Sacred Geometry - Philosophy and Practice) Thames and Hudson 1982

Gyorgy Doczi (The Power of Limits - Proportional Harmonies in Nature, Art and Architecture) Shambala Publications 1981

R. A. Schwaller de Lubicz (The Temple in Man - Sacred Architecture and the Perfect Man) Autumn Press 1977

Masaru Emoto (The True Power of Water - Healing and discovering ourselves) Beyond Words 2005

Viktor Schauberger (The Water Wizard - The Extraordinary Properties of Natural Water) Gill 1999

J. Schwuchow, J. Wilkes et al. (Flowform Water Research 1970-2007) Healing Water Foundation 2008

A.M. Bell (Practical dowsing, A Symposium) G. Bell & Sons London 1965

Abbe Mermet (Principles and practice of Radiesthesia) Element Books 1987

Christian Braibant Archipuncture

Guy-Charles Ravier (Lecture orientale des sites et constructions d'occident par le « Feng-Shui » géographie et médecine populaire chinoise) CRES (Centre de Recherches sur l'Environnement de la Santé) Edition 1987

130

PHOTO CREDITS

Jean-Marie Gobet
Fremantle, Australia
12, 63, 79, 80, 81, 82

Martial Gobet
Romont, Switzerland
10, 11, 25, 48

Larry Hirshowitz
California, USA
41, 72, 105

Alesia Kozik
6

Kent Weakley
9

Elena11
14

taffpixture
17

muratart, PhotoVisions
18

Yaroslav Shuraev
20

Spiks
21

Sarazh Izmailov
22

Victor Lu
25

Morphart Creation
26, 27

Valente Romero
27

Harrison Candlin
28

F1lter 88
30

Helen Hotson
31

dies-irae
42

Waqas Saeed
49

Ana Benet
50

Giorgio G.
51

David Pineda Svenske.
52

Max Mishin
54

Alexey Fedorenko,
R_andrei
55

lightaspect
56

Pixabay, privetik
58

Mapics
61

Meggyn Pomerleau
63

Zita
66, 67

Nor Gal
68

ChameleonsEye
70

Osaze Cuomo
71

Giulio Fornasar
72

Hanna, Pixabay
74

eurooo, houzlook
75

Ryutaro Uozumi
76

Giulio Fornasar
72

DaiPhoto
77

Adwo
79

ShamAn77
81

Angelo Gilardelli
82

Alexandre Zveiger
83

ungvar
85

Beth Macdonald
86

Peeradontax,
Sebastien G.
87

Nadia Levinskaya
89

Peter Schreiber
90

Suriyachan
91

Tony Stoddard,
nobeastsofierce
92

Sucha Kittiwararat
93

PNW Production
95

Pixabay, mpix-foto,
Baimieng
97

Pixabay
98

Enrique
99

Nathan Hurst
100

J Mundy
102

Stockis
103

Mo Eid
104

Karen,
ArmadilloPhotograp
107

Skyler Ewing, Pixabay,
Chris G, Shane Myers
Photography
108

Jonathan Stutz
109, 117

Renata Sedmakova
115

Brad Pict
117

Tanya Maury
121

About the author:

After completing a 4-year architectural drafting apprenticeship at his uncle's architect's practice Swiss born Jean-Marie Gobet travelled around the world for 6 years during which time he worked for architects in Tahiti (French Polynesia) and Melaka (Malaysia). Jean-Marie then completed his architectural studies (B. Arch.) at the University of Western Australia in 1983.

In the mid-eighties he returned to work in Switzerland and studied the effects of sick building syndrome due to toxic materials and electromagnetic pollution, he then obtained a Diploma in Geobiology in France.

In the early nineties Jean-Marie lived in a community, in Northern Italy and then France where he participated in the design and construction of an eco-village at the "Domaine du Fan" between Limoges and Poitier.

Jean-Marie Gobet has more than forty years of experience in architecture, designing commercial, educational, medical, and residential buildings and is still practicing architecture in Fremantle WA.

"The Holistic House" is a summation of his experience offering solutions for a habitat that is not only healthy but an active contribution to one's physical and spiritual wellbeing.

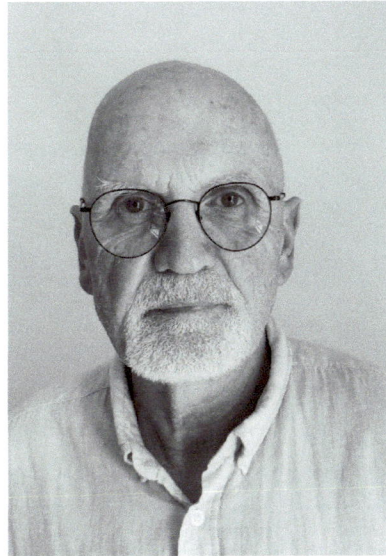

www.ingramcontent.com/pod-product-compliance
Lightning Source LLC
Chambersburg PA
CBHW041549030426

42334CB00005B/102